T0151083

DECODE
YOUR
DREAMS

IAN
WALLACE

DECODE
YOUR
DREAMS

UNLOCK YOUR
UNCONSCIOUS &
TRANSFORM YOUR
WAKING LIFE

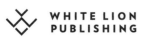
WHITE LION
PUBLISHING

TABLE OF CONTENTS

LOVE & SEX

RELATIONSHIPS & FAMILY

BIRTH & DEATH

WORK & PLAY

WEALTH & HEALTH

TRAVEL & DISCOVERY

PURPOSE & POTENTIAL

INTRODUCTION

For as long as humans have been dreaming, our dreams have been regarded as some largely indecipherable code. Various types of code-breaker emerged throughout the centuries of human existence. To begin with, they were fortune tellers and mystical seers, decoding what were generally considered to be messages from the gods. As human knowledge and understanding grew, more scientific methods were applied to the process of dream deciphering. In this approach, the human brain was considered to be a machine running code. The enigma of the dreaming brain was seen as a type of mechanistic computing engine and subsequently as an electronic computer.

The challenge with using the mystical or mechanistic approaches is that they are both largely ineffective in decoding the meaning of a dream. Both approaches make the assumption that dreaming is a passive process, with the dreamer simply observing what might be some etheric vibrations or random electrical brain noise. Towards the end of the twentieth century, more sophisticated brain-imaging techniques demonstrated that a dream was not just something that happened to you. In fact, the reverse was true. You actually happen to your dreams in the sense that you actively create everything that you experience in them.

The discovery that dreams are actively created with purpose and intention led to the realization that the person who might be trying to decode the dream is also the person who encoded it in the first place. Imaging studies had shown that specific areas of the brain were actively involved in creating a dream.

These areas included those concerned with emotional processing, need fulfilment, story generation and memory formation. Memories are experiences that hold meaning for you, so when you create a dream, you are encoding a meaningful story about how to fulfil your emotional needs in waking life.

Our word 'code' is derived from the word 'codex', originally meaning a significant and valuable book. The stories that you encode in your dreams are not just one-off events. They are your natural way of creating your own living book of who you are. The living book that you author in your dreams is not written in words. You tell it in vivid imagery and heartfelt emotions. You update that book of who you are every time you dream, and as you do so you are not just processing experiences of who you have been, but are also imagining the possibilities of who you can become.

Dreams are no longer some largely indecipherable code, and as you are the person encoding your dreams, you are the best person to decode them. In this book, you can learn how to decode your night-time dreams so that you can use that information to reflect on and resolve dilemmas, identify and release tensions, as well as to make your best dreams come true in your waking life.

HOW TO USE THIS BOOK

In the first part, 'The Power of Dreams', we explore the dreaming process and become more familiar with the significance and importance of dreams. This will help you to understand what dreams are, why we dream and what dreams mean. We also look at the difference between dreams and reality, and the fundamental link between dreams and emotions.

Next, we explore a range of universal dream themes and how to apply information from those themes to specific situations in your day-to-day life. It may seem as if using your dreams is a huge challenge because dream content is manifold, with billions and billions of variations. Happily, because we are all human beings and share many common behavioural patterns, we tend to create similar dream patterns and themes. Working with these dream themes is a useful way to make sense of the dreams that you create.

For each of the universal themes, there are a number of common dreams described. This book is not intended as a comprehensive dictionary. Instead, it is simply demonstrating the process of dream decoding by using examples that may be familiar to you. Each dream description provides a meaning for the dream, a waking-life action that corresponds to the dream and a question or prompt to help you put your dream into action. As you decode your dreams and understand what they mean, you will have the opportunity to turn the dreams that you create into positive and healthy action.

In 'Further Dreamwork', I then share some practical exercises for actively engaging with the dream imagery that you create, so that you can reconnect with its power and explore its potential in more depth. Lastly, we explore ways of turning your dreams into action in 'Make Your Dreams Come True', looking at how you can remember your dreams, what influences your dreams and how you can choose what happens in your dreams through lucid dreaming.

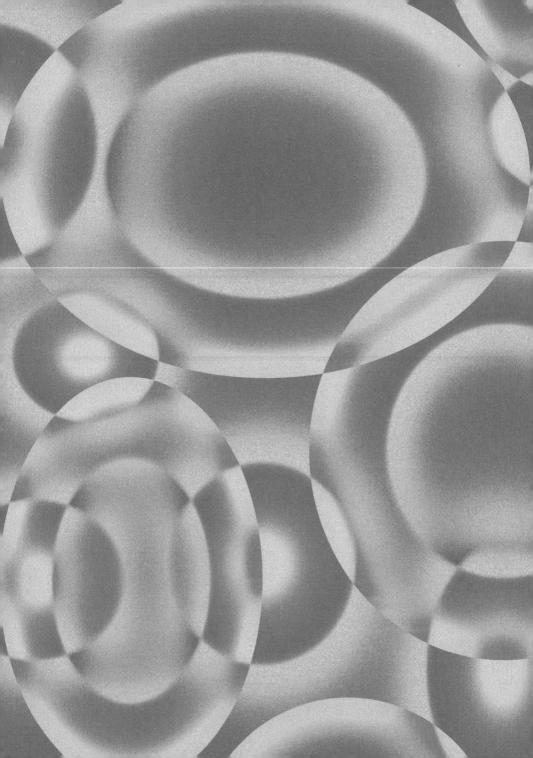

THE POWER OF DREAMS

Dreams can appear like fleeting, half-glimpsed experiences that have no real application in day-to-day life. Our dreams have the power to move us, to unsettle us, to inspire us, but using that power in waking life may seem a challenge. Understanding why you create the dreams that you do, however, naturally develops your human superpowers of self-awareness and situational awareness. The more aware you are of who you want to become and where you want to go in life, the more likely you are to succeed in doing so – and dreams are a doorway to doing just that.

We All Dream

Every human being dreams: every human being alive today, every human being who ever lived and every human being who will ever live. We humans have been fascinated by dreams since we first began communicating them and sharing them with each other.

The first written dream diaries date from more than 5,000 years ago in Nineveh on the banks of the Tigris, an ancient Assyrian city that forms part of modern-day Iraq. Dream dictionaries began to emerge around 2,000 years ago in ancient Greece and our fascination with dreams and the dreaming process continues into the twenty-first century.

Many misconceptions and superstitions about dreams have accumulated over those tens of thousands of years. Dreams were considered to be messages from the gods, communicating vital information if only we could work out what the messages meant. This belief deemed human beings as some type of psychic receiver that was tuning into the realm of the gods, who were actively sending out messages to be passively received by the dreaming humans.

During the twentieth century, equipment for measuring electrical activity in the brain became more widely available. As a result, scientists began to oppose the belief that dreams were messages from the gods, and instead proposed that dreams did not mean anything and were just random electrical activity in the brain.

Towards the end of the twentieth century, brain researchers and psychologists discovered that dreams were being actively created by the brain, rather than passively experienced, and this led to renewed interest in the idea that dreams actually might mean something. Researchers started considering dream images as components of a language instead of dismissing them as superstitions or electrical neuron noise.

In this linguistic approach, the images in dreams began to be studied from a metaphorical perspective. Up until that point, metaphors had typically been considered merely to be a form of language ornamentation. Advances in cognitive linguistics, however, demonstrated that conceptual thought processes have a largely metaphorical basis. A metaphor is a figure of speech that uses one thing to represent another thing, like using 'crazy about you' to symbolize a seemingly uncontrollable attraction. In both our dreams and in our waking lives, we use the 'whats' of our everyday experiences metaphorically, to represent the 'whys' of our conceptual processes.

Dreams are no longer a mystery and now they can be used to solve the much bigger questions that every human encounters. And those questions are: who are you, who have you been and who can you become? You are the person who can solve that mystery and the way you can do it is by decoding your dreams.

What Are Dreams?

A dream is how your brain makes sense of all the information and experiences that you unconsciously absorb every day in waking life. This individual sense-making process provides you with meaningful insights into specific challenges that you are encountering in your day-to-day life. Your dreams are not just a random occurrence; they are actually a deliberate process that you can use to draw on your past experience and help you understand ways to make the most of future opportunities.

From the perspective of a sleep scientist, the dreaming process is one of the main phases of the human sleeping cycle. Human beings tend to sleep in 90-minute cycles and you usually create dream episodes during each of these cycles.

In your first 90-minute sleep cycle, you will create dreams for about 10 to 15 minutes. During your last 90-minute sleep cycle before waking in the morning, you'll create dreams for about 40 to 45 minutes. On average, you will spend about two hours dreaming every night, which means that you spend a twelfth of your life dreaming.

Phase 1

The first phase of sleep in the cycle is light sleep, when you may create some imagery as you relax and begin to drift off. These are known as hypnagogic hallucinations and usually take the form of apparently random flashes of imagery, often drawn from the day's events.

Phase 2

The second phase of sleep is deeper sleep and you will spend approximately half your sleeping time in phase two sleep in every 90-minute sleeping cycle.

Phase 3

The third phase of sleep is the deepest phase, during which your body repairs itself, restores your energy levels and boosts your immune system.

Phase 4

The fourth phase in a sleep cycle is the dreaming phase, also known as the Rapid Eye Movement or REM phase. Physically, the dreaming phase is characterized by rapidly moving eyes, increased breathing rate and significantly increased brain activity.

Why Do We Dream?

We dream as a way of continually updating our sense of self, so that we can understand who we actually are, what we really need and what we truly believe in our waking lives. Although you might spend some time thinking about your identity, needs and beliefs in waking life, you will usually only reflect on those aspects of yourself that you are consciously aware of. Self-reflection is a very positive and healthy process but, in waking life, at least 98 per cent of a person's self-awareness occurs at an unconscious level.

The 2 per cent in which a person is consciously aware is usually comprised of the physical and mental aspects of their waking life, particularly thoughts and ideas. The 98 per cent of unconscious awareness is largely comprised of the emotional and creative aspects of a person's self-awareness. One of the fundamental functions of dreaming is to process all the experiences and expectations that you unconsciously absorb every day. Every night, when you dream, you are sorting through all those experiences and expectations, moving the meaningful ones from your short-term memory into your long-term memory and letting go of those that no longer hold meaning for you.

Your brain processes these unconscious experiences and expectations in the form of imagery. Dreams are mainly visual images, as that is the most brain-intensive human sense, but your dreaming brain also uses sound, smell, taste and touch imagery. The imagery that you create every night in your dreams is a powerful and healthy reflection of how you see yourself at a deeper and more authentic level. When you dream, you are exploring how you see yourself in your waking life so that you can imagine who you can become.

Imagery in Dreams

Although your dreams naturally help you identify what is most significant for you in your waking life, they can often seem like a meaningless stream of random imagery. The key to decoding your dreams is to identify why those images are important to you so that you can make sense of what they represent to you in real life.

The most practical way to decode your dream images is to begin by understanding the connection between what the dream image represents and why that is significant in your waking life. It will help if you first recognize that different types of dream imagery equate to different aspects of yourself or waking-life situations you are experiencing.

As you make these connections between your dream life and your real life, look out for metaphors as well. For example, if you create a dream where you are climbing a mountain, try connecting that to a specific situation in your waking life that might seem to be 'an uphill struggle' or in which you 'have a mountain to climb'. Dreaming of pregnancy suggests that you have a 'labour of love' that you want to bring into existence. A dream of losing your car can indicate a loss of 'drive' and 'motivation'.

Here are some key examples:

- When you create the dream image of a **person**, for example, you are exploring an emerging awareness of a valuable aspect of your character. The quality that you associate most with that person is the characteristic that you can develop yourself.

- Similarly, creating a dream image of a **place** connects you to a specific situation in your waking life, one in which you have the personal resourcefulness to increase your awareness and self-worth.

- Dreaming of a particular **object**, meanwhile, connects you to an ability that you possess in real life, one that is ready to be used in your personal development.

- A dream image of an **event** is connecting you to an opportunity to take some positive and healthy action.

- Dream **animals** represent your instincts and creativity in real life so that you can solve problems using your experience and expertise.

- Dream images of **plants** are connecting you to your capacity for healthy and natural growth in waking life.

- Dreaming of parts of the **human body** symbolizes your fundamental power to take specific and decisive action in real life.

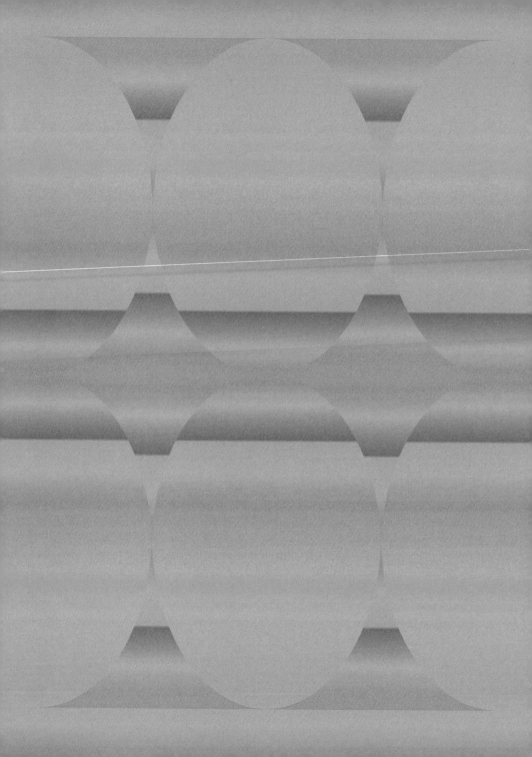

Dreams & Emotions

As your emotional life comprises a large part of your unconscious awareness, one of the main functions of dreaming is to process emotions and help to resolve any emotional tensions that you may be experiencing in waking life. Trying to process emotions can be quite difficult. Even when you are experiencing an intense emotion, it can be hard to put how you really feel into words. That's why, when we express our emotions in waking life, we tend to use linguistic imagery such as idioms and metaphors. If a person is angry, for example, it is quite rare for them to simply state 'I am angry'. They are far more likely to use a linguistic image such as 'I am utterly fuming about that decision' or 'If he does that again, I will absolutely erupt'.

In the same way that we use linguistic images to express our emotions in waking life, we also use imagery in our dreams as a way of processing our emotions. Your dreams are not just a stream of images, they are also a flow of emotions. The more powerful the emotions are that you are processing, the more powerful the imagery will be that you create in your dreams. Although some of the dream images that you create might seem scary and overpowering, they are your brain's natural and healthy way of engaging with your deeper emotional power.

In waking life, you might find it challenging to resolve unspoken emotional tensions and work through deeper emotional issues. Your unconscious imagery is the natural language of your emotions and the images you create in your dreams give voice and form to emotional tensions so that you can successfully resolve them. As you engage more with your emotional power in your day-to-day life, you will also find yourself automatically developing your sense of self-awareness and situational awareness, opening you up to new possibilities and opportunities.

Dreams & Reality

One of the biggest challenges in decoding your dreams is understanding the difference between dreams and reality. Although you use elements and experiences from your real life as the basis for your dreams, your dreaming brain uses them in quite a different way than you consciously do in waking life. Everything that you encounter in real life has two fundamental aspects in the way that you perceive it. Those two aspects are what it is and why it is. Usually in waking life, the aspect we consciously focus on is the 'what': the utility and the functionality. Unconsciously, in real life, the aspect that really matters to us is the 'why': the meaning and the significance.

As your dreaming brain processes your waking-life experiences, it naturally works through what is most meaningful to you. Although you can consciously recognize what is physically and mentally meaningful to you in your waking life, it can be far more challenging to consciously work through what is emotionally and creatively significant to you.

When you create an image of something in your dreams, you are identifying why a specific quality in that thing holds some meaning for you rather than simply illustrates what the thing is. So when you create a dream of being inappropriately intimate with a work colleague – one who you have absolutely no attraction to in real life – you are actually identifying some quality associated with them that you find meaningful. That quality might be their confidence in dealing with challenging situations, their ability to help people feel at ease or perhaps something seemingly as trivial as their skill at making a great cup of coffee.

Decoding Your Dreams

When using a psychological approach to understand your dreams, the first step is to form a hypothesis about why you created particular imagery in your dream. Forming a hypothesis is how psychologists and scientists devise an initial explanation for some unexplained phenomenon. The word 'hypothesis' is derived from ancient Greek and means to 'place under', so it is the basic idea that supports your explanation. Dreams are flows of emotions as well as streams of imagery, so start forming your hypotheses by identifying the feelings that you experienced flowing under your dream imagery.

As you reflect on your dream imagery and the feelings flowing beneath it, you may find that you have a number of hypotheses you want to test. Begin with the one that you feel most drawn to. At this point, it can be tempting to jump to a conclusion, but remember, the imagery you created in your dream is symbolizing a 'why' from your waking life, rather than representing an actual 'what'. For example, if you dream that your partner is having an affair, then the literal interpretation is that your partner is being unfaithful. The symbolic interpretation, however, is that you are letting yourself down and betraying your talents in some way.

The best way to test your hypothesis is to reflect on the imagery that resonated most vividly with you in your dream. This is usually the symbol that holds most meaning for you and provides the underlying theme of the dream. Take that image and think about what it symbolically resembles in your waking life. So if you dream that you are naked in public, reflect on a situation in your day-to-day life where you might be feeling vulnerable and exposed. If you dream that you are falling, think about what might be good to let go of.

After identifying the underlying theme of the dream, consider the other imagery that you created in your dream and ask yourself whether it supports your hypothesis. For example, if you dream that you are naked in public and also trying to hide or cover yourself up in the dream, that would support your hypothesis that you feel vulnerable in waking life and are trying to hide or cover up your embarrassment. After you have established a hypothesis that makes sense and feels right for you, the next step is to turn your dream into action.

A dream is just a dream until you turn it into action and you do that by consciously asking yourself the question that the dream is unconsciously answering for you. So if you dream of being naked in public, then the action would be to open up and reveal more of your authentic self in a situation in which you feel vulnerable and exposed in waking life. The question that would get you to action might be 'When can you be more open about displaying your knowledge and experience to others rather than feeling vulnerable to their potential criticism?'

You may find that answers are not surfacing for you straight away, so just take time to reflect on the question and see what answers emerge. It is always useful to notice your initial reaction to your question and see how that might change after you have considered your question for a while. You may feel that it is not the right time to take any action, but through the process of asking yourself the question, you have opened up some possible choices. The questions that emerge from your dreams are the questions that reveal your conversation with your future self, the person you have the power to become.

Quick Guide to Creating a Dream Hypothesis

Begin with the image from your dream that
resonates most strongly with you.

———○———

Relate the dream image to your waking life –
what could it represent?

———○———

Think about the other images from your dream –
do they fit your hypothesis?

———○———

What question from your waking life might
your dream be answering?

———○———

See if you can put the question into
words or a drawing.

———○———

Take your time to reflect on your
question and see what answers emerge.

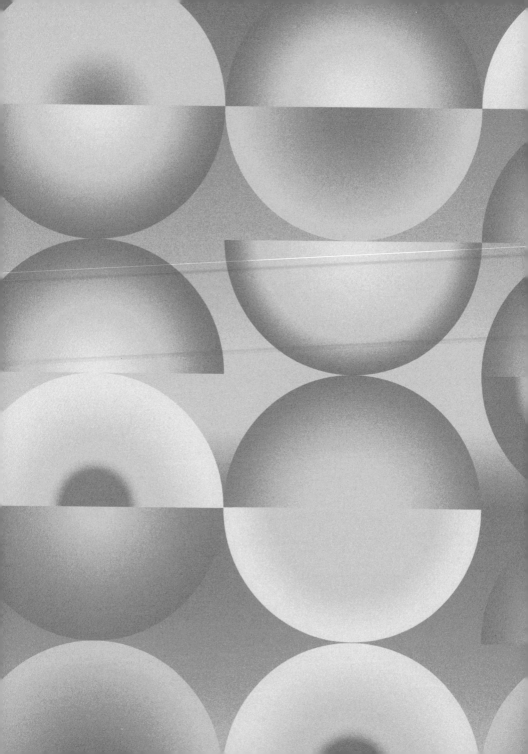

LOVE
& SEX

Dreams are how we process all the emotions we experience in our day-to-day lives. Emotions associated with our love and sex lives are among the most intense that we feel. We use our dreams not only to work through our waking experiences of love and sex but also to explore the significance of love and sex at a much deeper level. When we dream, we use love to symbolize what we love most in the outer world and what we love most about ourselves in our inner world. Sexual imagery symbolizes our talent for conceiving and creating what we desire in our waking lives.

In this chapter, you will discover the significance of how you express your deeper desires in different dream scenarios: why sex dreams are not really about sex, how creativity is connected to making love in our dreams, the difference between love and sex dreams and what your dream lover can reveal about your creative potential. To take your love and sex dream work further, try the exercise on page 170.

Love Dreams

Love dreams are a way of creating a deeper understanding of what you desire most in life. Although these dreams may feature a specific lover, such as someone you know, the lovers in your dreams actually symbolize creative ideas or activities that you are passionate about. We can find ourselves being irresistibly drawn towards exciting issues and ideas in daily life, just as we might be drawn to a lover. However, even though you may have set your heart on a perfect outcome, following your true desire can be challenging.

Secret crush

UNLOCK THE MEANING

Dreaming about a secret crush may seem like unrequited wish fulfilment, but creating this dream indicates a growing awareness of a dormant talent that you possess. The secret crush symbolizes your attraction towards a particular plan or activity that you feel passionate about. Your hurdles are self-doubt and pride: what if you are not good enough or lack talent? Will your creative ideas and actions be rejected by other people? Rather than opening yourself up and risking criticism or ridicule, it can seem easier to fantasize about your secret talent and not take action.

AWAKEN YOUR POTENTIAL

Find strength in discovering your passions and thrill in their possibilities. Embrace your potential and confidently demonstrate your talent to others. Discover that making the commitment to this talent, and engaging with it, will be a fulfilling experience. It may become what you love doing most in your life. Even if it feels like others are pushing back, continue to commit and persevere. You will find joy in the advances you make.

The time you spend doing what you love most can be limited by other commitments or obligations. An opportunity to reconnect with a neglected or former passion may be represented in a dream by a first love or returning lover.

First love

UNLOCK THE MEANING

A first love appearing in a dream symbolizes an idea or an activity that was once a favourite pastime, perhaps one that you lovingly dedicated much time to and took great enjoyment from. Although you may have moved on to developing other talents, that first love often remains a fundamental passion of yours.

AWAKEN YOUR POTENTIAL

Take some time to reflect on what initially inspired you to pursue that first passion. You may feel that you have moved on, but you now have the opportunity to reconnect with it and to develop it further. Pause and reflect on whether you wish to connect with what originally inspired you or you are happy to acknowledge it but leave it in the past.

As you continue to develop your talents beyond your initial passions, you can build the confidence to engage with a range of activities and ideas that you are enthusiastic about. Reconnecting with a specific idea or activity is often reflected in a dream where a lover returns.

Return of an ex-lover

UNLOCK THE MEANING

Dreaming of a returning lover shows that you are becoming aware of an exciting opportunity in your waking life, one in which you can reconnect with an interest or pursuit that you were once very keen on. The time is now. The challenge is deciding whether you want to do that or not.

AWAKEN YOUR POTENTIAL

Consider the implications of reconnecting with an interest or pursuit that you previously felt passionate about. Rather than being inevitably drawn towards it again, you can now choose if you want to revive this interest or not. Making this decision will help you to find clarity on what is meaningful and exciting to you at the present time.

Love dreams reflect what you feel most excited about in your waking life and your commitment to channelling your energies into that passion. Just as in a relationship, you may sometimes question your ability to remain committed and in a dream this feeling may be portrayed as an affair.

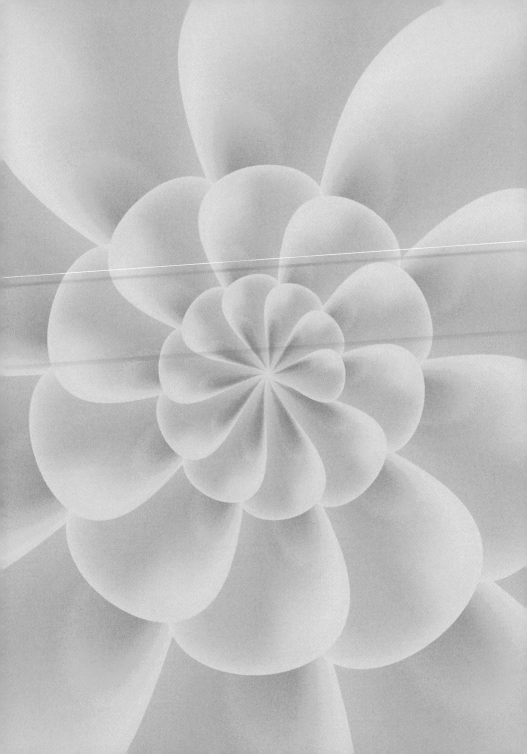

Having an affair

UNLOCK THE MEANING

Dreaming that you or your partner are having an affair has nothing to do with being unfaithful in waking life. Rather, this dream reflects a situation in which you feel guilty for letting yourself down; you are betraying your commitment to a creative process or activity that is close to your heart. You have lost self-confidence and faith in your abilities and this, in turn, is preventing you from reaching your potential.

AWAKEN YOUR POTENTIAL

Believe in your natural talents and abilities and be proud of what your passion has helped you to create so far. Rather than investing energy in feeling guilty about letting yourself down, make the commitment to develop your capabilities confidently. It may be that you have faith in your talents but worry that other people will disapprove of your passion and try to stop you pursuing it. This passion is a fundamental part of who you are, so have the courage to defend it.

If other people describe your pursuit as irrational and you try to please them by ignoring your passion, it may show up in your dreams as an unconventional lover.

Unconventional lover

UNLOCK THE MEANING

An unconventional or irrational lover in your dreams means that your passion for a particular pursuit may be at odds with the rational self-image that you normally like to present to other people, so you feel compelled to restrain yourself from engaging with it under any circumstances.

AWAKEN YOUR POTENTIAL

Rather than feeling you have to contain your talents and your abilities by sticking to convention, consider unconventional approaches; sometimes a seemingly unrealistic idea might just work. In which situations can you use some creative thinking and a fresh new context for your talent to ensure a positive and healthy outcome without you losing sight of what is close to your heart?

If the lover in your dream is perfectly good company but not the right fit for you, then this is a dream of a wrong lover and may suggest that you are misdirecting your energies.

Wrong lover

UNLOCK THE MEANING

Dreaming of being with the wrong lover indicates that you are using your creativity and passion to achieve a successful outcome but your heart is not really in what you are doing. The dream lover may appear to be rational and easy to connect with, but you know deep down that they are not the right lover for you. They just don't excite your passions or give you the inspiration that you desire. This usually reflects a waking-life situation in which you are using your creative energies to please another person.

AWAKEN YOUR POTENTIAL

Instead of focusing your energies on helping someone else to achieve their ambitions, channel your talents into working towards something that you truly desire for yourself. Ask yourself how you might use your creative passion to fulfil your own desires rather than just simply using your talents to fulfil the desires of other people. Although it is always gratifying to feel useful, try to maintain a positive and healthy balance of how you direct your energies between your own desires and those of others.

Contrastingly, a lover in your dreams may seem absolutely right for you but mysterious or elusive, and this can reveal a wish to exert more control over your talents.

Mystery lover

UNLOCK THE MEANING

If a seemingly perfect lover recurrently appears in your dreams but disappears just as you begin to feel really close to them, it indicates that you view your creative abilities as talents that just come and go, rather than being able to call on them when you need them. In waking life, a mysterious lover can seem very attractive because you always want to find out more about them. In a dream, a mysterious lover suggests that you are keen to find out how to consistently engage with your talent.

AWAKEN YOUR POTENTIAL

Take a more structured approach to how you employ your creative talents, so that you can apply them as soon you need them, instead of simply waiting for inspiration to strike. Think about how you can create a consistent and repeatable framework to support you as you channel your creativity into your passion project. For example, when learning a new skill, it can often seem like a complete mystery to begin with, even if you have a natural aptitude for it. Structuring your learning process helps you learn more effectively, and the same is true when you are developing a talent.

Sex
Dreams

Whereas love dreams reflect your irresistible attraction to ideas and activities that you feel passionate about in waking life, sex dreams are all about embracing and embodying those waking-life passions. You will often find yourself conceiving new ideas as your creative juices start to flow. As you do so, you may find yourself opening up more about your ideas to others, and, equally, being more receptive to the ideas that other people are offering you. This can result in an intertwining of ideas and activities that might have initially seemed quite different to each other. The more intimately aware you become of the nature of this creative process, the more intimately aware you become of your unique talents.

Passionate kissing

UNLOCK THE MEANING

In dreams your mouth symbolizes how confident you feel about being able to express honestly what you desire most in your waking life. Your lips and tongue represent your ability to do this in a sensitive and tasteful manner. Although the person you are kissing in the dream may have some symbolic significance, this dream is really about forming a deeper connection with yourself. The most important information from this dream is that you are realizing that you have the ability to clearly articulate what you desire most, rather than just blurt it out in a tasteless and insensitive manner.

AWAKEN YOUR POTENTIAL

Rather than remaining tight-lipped about an idea that you feel deeply drawn to, have the confidence to speak up. For example, you may feel passionate about studying drama at university but lack confidence in yourself or feel other people do not support your aim. Having the conviction to declare your passion and commit to it often attracts the support that may have been lacking. Think about how you might sensitively communicate your deeper feelings and openly express your passion. Remember to be receptive when others voice their own desires so that you can combine your creative energies and work together towards a mutually satisfactory result.

Passionate kissing in a dream often leads to greater intimacy with a dream partner, even though they may not be an intimate partner you would choose in waking life.

Intimacy with an unlikely partner

UNLOCK THE MEANING

An intimate partner in your dream is not a direct representation of that person in waking life. Instead, they are your dreaming brain's way of characterizing particular qualities. A dream lover is often someone who you know in waking life and believe to possess a specific quality. They might also be a composite of a number of people that you have identified as having that characteristic quality. An unlikely partner in a dream indicates an opportunity to develop a particular talent that may seem unfamiliar to you. Whatever quality you associate most with that person is the quality that you now have the opportunity to use in a positive and healthy manner.

AWAKEN YOUR POTENTIAL

Consider the quality that you associate most with your dream partner. If, for example, they are brimming with confidence, aspire to have more confidence in your own talents and experiences in your day-to-day activities. Ask yourself how you might use that talent to make the most of an opportunity.

As well as creating dreams in which you are being intimate with an unlikely partner, you may also dream of having sex in an unusual place. While the first symbolizes a particular quality, the unfamiliar location reflects a particular situation.

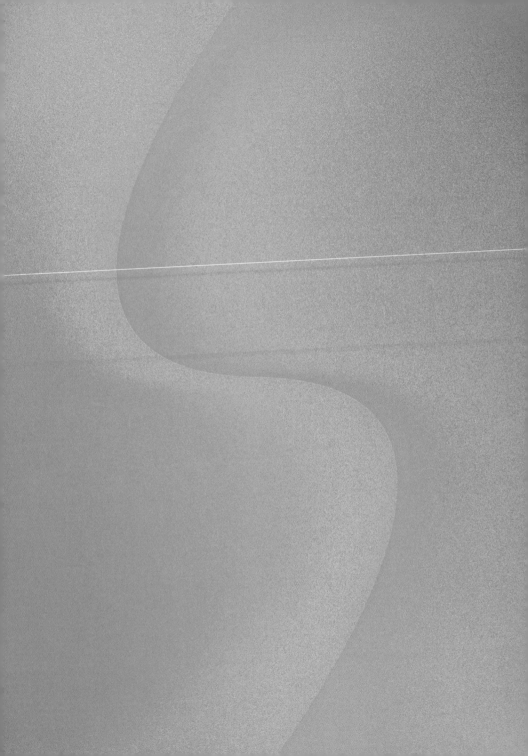

Sex in an unusual place

UNLOCK THE MEANING

Places in dreams represent particular situations in your waking life. Dreaming of sex in an unusual location suggests that an unusual situation has arisen in your day-to-day life. This new circumstance is providing you with a golden opportunity to use your creative talents and passion in a fresh context, one that may be unnervingly unfamiliar.

AWAKEN YOUR POTENTIAL

Challenge yourself to be strategic. Investigate how you might use your creative drive and passion to make the most of an opportunity. Even though you may feel out of place in these new circumstances, know that this is the time to let your talent shine through. For example, say you write a personal blog about a subject that you feel excited about and then find yourself being invited to write an article for a prestigious international magazine – this dream is urging you to take up the opportunity.

Dreaming of forbidden sexual practices can be unsettling, but we always have to remember that dreams and reality are quite different. Sexual acts in dreams don't actually represent those in waking life, but instead help us to identify different methods of using our creative passions.

Forbidden sex

UNLOCK THE MEANING

Dreaming of engaging in forbidden sexual practices suggests that you feel you are being prevented from developing a particular creative talent in your waking life. This is often caused by those who are jealous of your growing skills and who take a perverse pleasure in attempting to limit your advancement, but it can also be that you are limiting your own ambitions.

AWAKEN YOUR POTENTIAL

A simple antidote to self-imposed limitations is self-trust and openness. Give yourself permission to explore some of the less conventional areas of your creative talents. Although this may simply feel like indulging in a guilty pleasure, it will enable you to expand your skills beyond what you had previously sanctioned or expected of yourself, and will help you break free from the limitations placed on you by other people. This will give you space to allow more positive opportunities to present themselves.

While a forbidden sex dream indicates a sense that your creative development is being stunted by the choices of other people, you may also create dreams that do not reflect your sexual preferences in your waking life.

New sexual preference

UNLOCK THE MEANING

Sex dreams can be both unsettling and exciting, especially when they offer glimpses into sexual practices that you may not choose to indulge in waking life. When you dream of being intimate with a partner in way that is outside your waking-life sexual preference, it suggests that you may be taking quite a fixed approach to developing one of your creative talents. This can result in you becoming absorbed in a specific method of problem-solving, which then narrows your creative options.

AWAKEN YOUR POTENTIAL

Think about the situations in which you need to be more open to different creative methods. Although you may feel that there is a best way to solve a particular problem, there may be other ways that will be equally as effective and potentially lead to more creative opportunities and choices. Fixating on the one that you routinely use may prove counterproductive.

Remember that just as unusual sexual practices and partner preferences are not representative of literal waking-life desires, dreaming of being simultaneously intimate with multiple partners does not mean that you actually want to do that in real life.

At an orgy

UNLOCK THE MEANING

Actively participating in a dreamed orgy indicates an opportunity in waking life to share your creative talents with a wider variety of other people. Although you may not conceive any new ideas with them, it will expand your understanding of the range of creative processes used by others.

AWAKEN YOUR POTENTIAL

Embrace greater openness to the creative ideas of others, even if your natural choice might be to focus on one idea and work through it in greater depth. Find space to display your creative talents and problem-solving skills to people with whom you might not normally engage. Give yourself permission to draw on inspiration from others and collaborate with them rather than feel that you have to create everything yourself.

In an orgy dream, you may experience a loss of identity and a lack of intimacy, perhaps feeling anonymous with nothing special to identify your unique talents. This same sensation can emerge when you dream of being sexually intimate with a faceless partner whom you cannot seem to identify.

Faceless partner

UNLOCK THE MEANING

When you dream, a person's face always symbolizes some aspect of your identity, so dreaming of a faceless sexual partner shows that you are finding it challenging to identify an important part of your creative process and talent in waking life. This can often happen because you lack confidence in your skills and may be trying to keep your contributions anonymous.

AWAKEN YOUR POTENTIAL

Rather than worrying about somehow losing face if you display your creative skills to other people, face up to the fact that you have great talent and know that, as you continue to develop it, you will naturally begin to identify your own unique style and voice. Trying to be humble can often be a form of false modesty, so choose to be true to your talents. Consider how you can bring your solution-savvy skills to the attention of other people, both to assist them and to work towards making the most of your strengths.

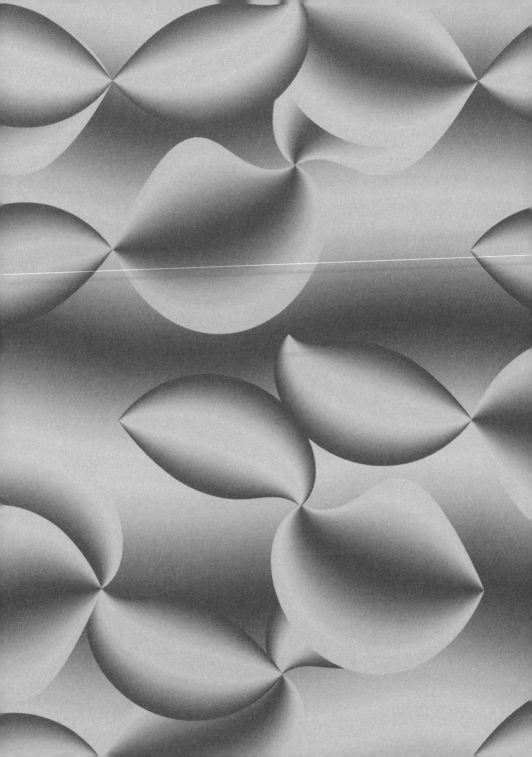

RELATIONSHIPS
& FAMILY

You may think of yourself as having a single identity, the one described by your name, in your passport or in your online presence. The psychological reality, however, is that you have a number of identities. This is not some sort of split personality; your different identities emerge depending on the circumstances you find yourself in and the actions you take there. For example, your job title may be CEO but in a single day, you could also be a driver, a passenger and a customer, and also a mother, a wife and a sister.

In this chapter, you will learn the significance of how you relate to your family and others in different dream scenarios, and discover why relationship dreams are not really about relationships, how family dreams are connected to habitual behaviours, the difference between relationships and family dreams, and what your relationship dreams can reveal about your potential for personal development. To take your relationship and family dream work further, try the exercise on page 170.

Relationship Dreams

Although our love and sex partnerships may seem to take priority in our waking lives, we also have important relationships in the form of our friendships, and these can be even more significant and enduring. When you dream, you use the people in your relationships to symbolize the emotional qualities that you associate with them. For example, if the characteristic quality that you associate with a particular friend is compassion, then you would use that friend in your dream to represent that quality. You do that because you have an opportunity in your waking life to develop and display your sense of compassion.

Getting married

UNLOCK THE MEANING

Dreaming of getting married does not necessarily mean that someone is about to pop the question or you are having pre-wedding nerves in waking life. It actually suggests that you are thinking about a major commitment or decision, one in which you are trying to balance different obligations, such as your work life and your family life. A marriage symbolizes a serious commitment that is intended to last for life.

AWAKEN YOUR POTENTIAL

Take some time to reflect on the day-to-day activities that you are engaged in and the commitments that you are involved in. How can you achieve a better balance in your commitments to other people without neglecting your own needs? Although you may have to be open to making some compromises, remember to honour your commitments to yourself as well as others.

In a marriage, we have one special person with whom we share love and support. Beyond that relationship, we also have a wider supporting cast of friends, as well as a whole range of people that we know and perhaps look up to, such as celebrities, who may appear in our dreams.

Celebrity friend

UNLOCK THE MEANING

Dreaming of being friends with a celebrity is not merely some form of wishful fulfilment. A celebrity represents a public display of potentially valuable and attractive characteristics. The celebrity in your dream indicates that you have the opportunity to attract more people to your way of thinking and demonstrate the value of your talents.

AWAKEN YOUR POTENTIAL

How might you attract more people to your way of thinking? By having the confidence to publicly display your talents and experience to them. You may feel shy about displaying your talent because other people may criticize it out of jealousy or because it doesn't conform to their worldview. Rather than feeling rejected by others, you might find it easier to conceal your talent and continue to be accepted by them. The more that you accept and celebrate your own unique abilities, however the more likely it is that they will be accepted and valued by other people.

Our connection with celebrities are a form of one-way relationships, in which we can feel comfortable and familiar with their presence even though they may be unaware of ours. Our real-life friendships, meanwhile, are two-way relationships that offer mutual trust and understanding.

Meeting an old friend

UNLOCK THE MEANING

When you dream of meeting an old friend, even one from many, many years ago, it shows that you are becoming reacquainted with the quality that you most associate with that person. An old friend appearing in your dream indicates that you have the opportunity to use that quality to resolve a challenge in your current circumstances.

AWAKEN YOUR POTENTIAL

Might you need to reacquaint yourself with a particular skill that you have not had the opportunity to use for a while? Take your time reconnecting with this talent or achievement that you may forgotten about. At first, it may seem a little awkward getting used to it again, but you'll soon feel at ease with displaying your capabilities. For example, your friend may have always been able to keep a cool head in a crisis and rationally work out the best way to resolve a dilemma. You now have the opportunity to use that characteristic coolness yourself and work out the best solution to a challenge that you are facing.

If you feel that you might be in danger of losing the opportunity to reacquaint yourself with a particular skill, then you may dream of trying to rescue a friend rather than just meeting them.

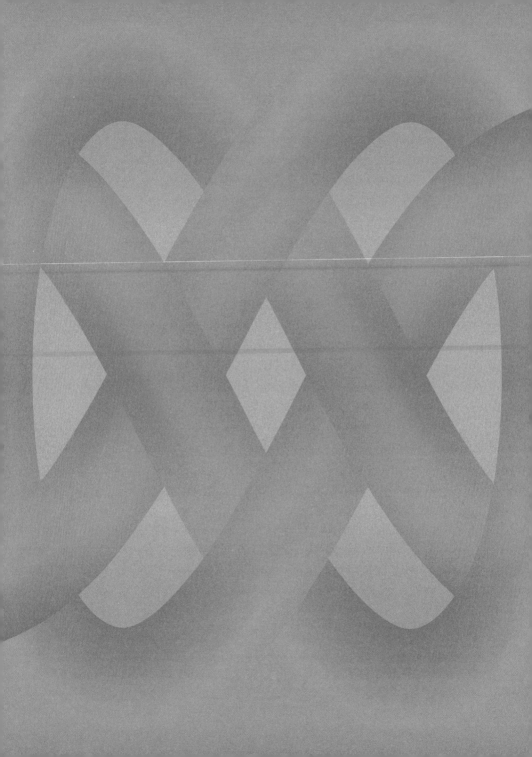

Rescuing a friend

UNLOCK THE MEANING

Rescuing a friend in a dream, often from a scenario where they are at risk of being lost forever, suggests that you have a valuable talent or skill that you feel you may not have the opportunity to use again, but that you are driven to save. The characteristic quality that you associate with the friend you are rescuing in the dream is the one that you need to reconnect with in order to save yourself from losing it.

AWAKEN YOUR POTENTIAL

Rather than allowing your proficiency in a valuable skill to fade away, make sure you maintain it by creating the time and space to regularly practise it. That skill might be a learned talent that enables you to express yourself in a unique way, such as playing a musical instrument, or it might be the ability to speak persuasively about an issue that you feel strongly. This is something that may help you in the future; although practising your talent may require some discipline, it will give you greater freedom in deciding your future.

If instead of trying to rescue one friend in your dream you find yourself trying to lead many or being involved in some kind of war, then this may point to some conflicting needs in your waking life, such as occasions when you have been trying to keep the peace.

Caught up in a war

UNLOCK THE MEANING

Dreaming of being caught up in a war suggests that you are trying to navigate your way through some conflicting circumstances in waking life. Potentially damaging tensions may arise because you may have to resolve things forcefully. The conflict may be between your own needs, or between your needs and those of other people. In this dream, you may feel personally responsible for a safe outcome and you may also feel that you are the only person who can ensure a positive and healthy conclusion.

AWAKEN YOUR POTENTIAL

In what situations do you need to confront your conflicting feelings so that you can successfully resolve any tensions you may be experiencing? The most effective way to resolve any conflict within yourself or with others is to be really clear about what you need. The more that you try to escape and evade conflict, the more likely that any internal battles will rumble endlessly on.

Sometimes relationship tensions are not so threatening and obvious that you create dreams of actual warfare. Often you may feel like others are invading your personal time and space with little respect for your boundaries.

Uninvited guests

UNLOCK THE MEANING

If you dream of uninvited guests intruding into one of your personal spaces, this reflects a waking-life situation in which you feel that you are being distracted from pursuing a personal ambition. It may seem as if you are unable to prevent these unwelcome distractions, but you are actually reminding yourself that you can maintain your focus by establishing personal boundaries.

AWAKEN YOUR POTENTIAL

Have the grace and courage to say 'no' as a way of establishing your own limits and boundaries. It may seem easier and more friendly to simply say 'yes' to every request for your help in your day-to-day life, but saying 'yes' all the time to other people means that you are habitually saying 'no' to your own needs. Review your scheduled commitments and consider how you might claim more time for yourself, your individual priorities and desires – rather than always feeling distracted by what other people need from you. This can be a challenge, but it will also open up new possibilities.

Sometimes you may need to release yourself from obligations that you agreed to in different circumstances. While those commitments may have made sense at the time you made them, you now feel that you can no longer honour them.

Getting divorced

UNLOCK THE MEANING

Even if you are in a happy and fulfilling marriage in your waking life, you may still dream of getting divorced. This dream has nothing to do with actual divorce proceedings. A divorce symbolizes a situation in which you feel you are having to committing too much time and effort to a particular obligation in your waking life and want to release yourself from it.

AWAKEN YOUR POTENTIAL

Have you forgotten to prioritize your own development over those of others? Spend some time thinking about your commitment to your own personal growth and fulfilment rather than being tied down by obligations to others. This does not mean you have to abandon all your commitments to other people. You just have to create a healthy balance with your own needs.

Family Dreams

Our earliest experiences of relationships are with our family members. In the same way that we use our wider relationships to characterize specific qualities, we also use our family relationships, particularly for qualities that are familiar and habitual. Family dreams give you the opportunity to explore and understand the different characters that you embody, such as your inner child and your older, wiser self. In waking life, we also associate our homes with our families and so we use the home as a way of symbolizing where we feel most comfortable.

Childhood home

UNLOCK THE MEANING

In dreams a house symbolizes your identity. Dreaming about your childhood house indicates that you are revisiting the origins of your identity and all the potential you have for future development. Although you may feel your identity is now fully formed, the childhood house suggests that you still have the opportunity to grow.

AWAKEN YOUR POTENTIAL

Take some time to reflect on the ideas and influences that have shaped your identity so far in your life. Think about who you can still become and give yourself permission to start playing around with a skill or interest that you have wanted to develop all your life.

A childhood home represents the origins of your identity and all your potential for future development. But a child in a dream symbolizes something slightly different: your potential for developing a plan or idea that is close to your heart.

Children in jeopardy

UNLOCK THE MEANING

Dreaming that your children are in some form of jeopardy is not a premonition that they are going to be in actual danger. The child or children in your dream represent a waking-life plan or an idea that is very precious to you, one that you are trying to nurture lovingly. Your concern is that the successful development of this plan is under some type of threat.

AWAKEN YOUR POTENTIAL

Give yourself permission to devote more time to developing the idea or plan that is close to your heart. Although the threat to your plan may seem to come from external influences, the main danger is that you are not devoting enough time to it. Ask yourself when you can find this time, and once you have identified this, protect that space. Not paying plans enough attention can put them in peril.

_____

At other times, we realize that we have been neglecting a plan or pursuit that was once very meaningful for us. This fear might materialize in a dream as an abandoned baby.

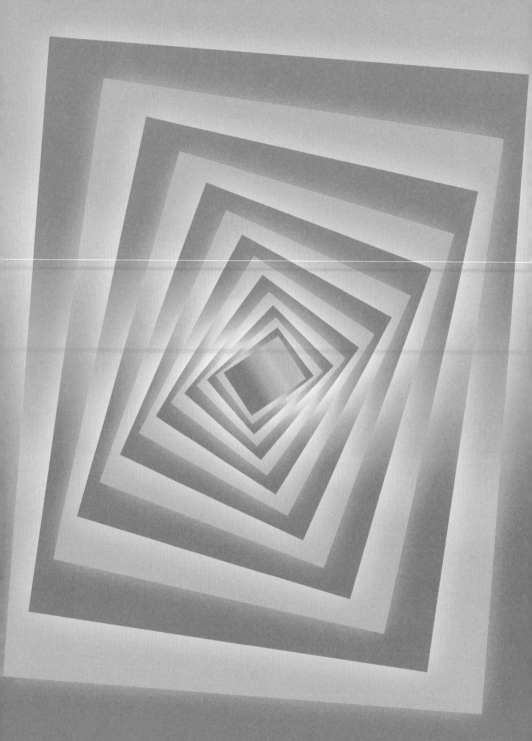

Abandoned baby

UNLOCK THE MEANING

If you dream about finding an abandoned baby, it suggests that you have the opportunity to reconnect with an idea or activity that was once very important to you but which you had to abandon for some reason. Because of your previous circumstances, you had to lay these ambitions to one side in the hope that you could continue to develop them at some point in the future.

AWAKEN YOUR POTENTIAL

Devote some of your resources to progressing an idea or ambition that was once very precious to you. It may seem easier to ignore your deeper needs, but this ambition will keep crying out for your attention until you take the time to develop it. Act decisively and swiftly on this instinct to avoid this abandoned ambition becoming a recurring concern. What other steps can you take to pursue your reignited passion?

We have a fundamental need to take care of a precious life that seems vulnerable and may not continue to exist without our immediate attention. As well as being true of our need to nurture our babies, it is also true of our need to look after our pets.

Neglected pet

UNLOCK THE MEANING

Pets are often considered to be part of a family. Dreaming of a family pet is how you symbolize your instinctive and creative nature. Encountering a neglected pet in your dream indicates that you have been disregarding this part of yourself, often because you feel you have to hide your true feelings so that you can peacefully get along with other people. Being unable to give voice to your emotions, however, can result in you feeling starved of affection by the people closest to you.

AWAKEN YOUR POTENTIAL

Speak up and clearly voice your needs to the people closest to you. Selflessly caring for others may lead to you feeling taken for granted. Remind others how much care and attention you give to them and gently seek their reciprocal attention. Consider how different types of pets and their attributes symbolize different aspects of your instinctive nature and, in turn, your needs. For example, dogs represent your need for loyalty and affection, and cats represent your requirement for comfort and independence.

Communicating our needs to loved ones can be challenging because we fear the possibility of an unwelcome reaction. Although we may have been trying to make our relationship better, we may worry that telling our loved ones what we really need might make a relationship worse.

Angry parent

UNLOCK THE MEANING

A parent symbolizes a fundamental sense of security and the authority to develop your potential as a person lovingly. Dreaming of being involved in an angry confrontation with a parent indicates that you feel conflicted about developing this aspect of your potential because you feel you need the permission of others to proceed.

AWAKEN YOUR POTENTIAL

Rather than feeling resentful that no one is giving you permission to proceed, take responsibility for your own actions and potential. When you reflect on your own self-judgements, inner conflicts and self-jeopardization strategies, you are less likely to get involved in external conflicts with others. As an act of self-care and self-kindness, think about those times when you need to give yourself approval to develop some aspect of your unique potential. It may seem selfish to look after your own needs before the needs of others, but that is misguided.

A deep-rooted sense of obligation can result in a situation in which you feel that others are making unfair demands on your time and resources. This leads to a frustration that can be dreamed as a kidnap scenario.

Kidnapped by a gang

UNLOCK THE MEANING

Being kidnapped by a gang in a dream can indicate that you feel forced into doing things that you would rather not do in waking life. This can often happen in family situations in which other family members seem to be trying to control your actions and ambitions in some way.

AWAKEN YOUR POTENTIAL

Take full responsibility for your own decisions. You can still be loyal to your family, but the more responsibly you behave, the less likely it is that you will feel trapped through seeking the approval of your family members. In which situations can you feel more accountable to yourself instead of always trying to meet the expectations of your family?

Doing what others expect of you against your own inclinations can result in a situation in which you feel that you are losing your sense of self. As your home symbolizes where you feel most comfortable, you may dream that you can't find your way home.

Can't find your way home

UNLOCK THE MEANING

Dreaming that you can't find your way home reflects a situation in your waking life in which you are doing what others want in order to seek their approval or affection. This can give you a false sense of security, as you are accommodating the needs of others in the hope that they will, in turn, accommodate your needs.

AWAKEN YOUR POTENTIAL

Rather than always allowing others to determine the direction you take, have the confidence to choose your own path in life. Clearly expressing your needs to other people is the best way to feel at home within yourself and comfortable with who you are. Feeling independent will prove a vital foundation for regaining your sense of self. Making your own decisions, such as choosing the food that you eat or the clothes that you wear, is the key to building your sense of independence.

BIRTH
& DEATH

Births and deaths are among the most profound events that we experience in our waking lives. When we dream, we use those intense experiences to represent significant beginnings and endings in our waking lives. Dreaming of birth and pregnancy reflects a situation in your waking life in which you are experiencing a new beginning. Dreams of death and dying symbolize the ending of some activity, a time when you are leaving behind what no longer nourishes you so that you can step into fresh new opportunities. As you do so, you will find yourself beginning anew, as the natural cycle continues.

In this chapter, you will discover the significance of how you explore potential opportunities in different dream scenarios: why death dreams are never really about death, how starting something new is connected to giving birth, the difference between birth and death dreams and why birth and death dreams are part of a natural growth cycle. To take your birth and death dream work further, try the exercise on page 171.

Birth Dreams

Birth dreams indicate that something new and exciting is emerging in your waking life. Like any birth event, this new beginning is the outcome of the seed of an idea that you may have conceived some time ago. Births don't just happen: they are the result of nurturing a precious conception and bringing it to a successful fruition. In the same way, the beginning of an exciting new stage in your life is often the fruit of previous labours over a period of time. As you bring your labour of love into the world, you naturally open up new opportunities for yourself.

Being pregnant

UNLOCK THE MEANING

Dreaming that you are pregnant often reflects a situation in your waking life in which you are taking a long time to nurture a concept or a plan into being. Although you may be very excited about the idea that you have conceived, you realize that there will be an extensive gestation period before you can bring it to life.

AWAKEN YOUR POTENTIAL

Do not rush; ensure that you develop your concept at a steady and natural pace. Even though you may be impatient to share your ideas with others, it is better not to bring them into the world prematurely. What projects of yours require time and nurturing in order to achieve a worthwhile outcome?

In contrast to this patiently developed end-goal process, you may dream of being constantly pregnant.

Endless pregnancy

UNLOCK THE MEANING

A dream in which you are constantly pregnant, with no indication of how long the pregnancy may last, suggests that you are holding on too tightly to an idea or ambition that you conceived a long while ago. Although other people may be offering you attractive inducements to produce your idea, you are concerned about the effort it may take.

AWAKEN YOUR POTENTIAL

Commit yourself to bringing your idea into the world. Even though you feel there may be a messy and challenging process ahead, it will turn your idea into reality. Consider the benefits of enjoying the rewarding conclusion of your efforts. You have the opportunity to create a uniquely wonderful outcome. What steps do you need to take to make one of your long-term plans happen?

Dreaming of the actual process of giving birth suggests that you now have the opportunity to bring that concept in life.

Giving birth

UNLOCK THE MEANING

Giving birth in a dream indicates that there is a situation in your waking life in which you can turn one of your ideas into practical reality, even though you may have conceived that idea quite a while ago. You have been carrying that idea around in your thoughts for some time and now you are realizing that the time is ripe to bring it into the world.

AWAKEN YOUR POTENTIAL

Realize that this long-term ambition may require a short period of serious effort and hard work. It may seem uncomfortable and intensely laborious at times, but the outcome will be worthwhile. You may also need to ask the help of others to facilitate the final push needed to turn what you have conceived into the outcome that you desire. Acknowledge the opportunity and the potential reward, make the commitment and persist.

Dreaming of having a difficult birth reflects a slightly different challenge: the difficulty of making one of your ideas an actual reality.

Difficult birth

UNLOCK THE MEANING

Being involved in a difficult birth in a dream suggests that you are meeting with lots of resistance in pushing your idea out to a wider audience. It seems like you are the only person who can make this happen, but that can be because you are cautious about asking for help.

AWAKEN YOUR POTENTIAL

Seeking assistance from other people is not a weakness. In fact, it is likely the best solution to your conundrum. You may feel that having other people involved will diminish your achievement, but that is misguided: you will still be the person who conceived the idea and brought it into the world.

If you experience the opposite type of birth in a dream, where you suddenly and unexpectedly give birth to a baby without any difficulty, a much easier path lies before you.

Unexpected birth

UNLOCK THE MEANING

Unexpectedly giving birth in a dream reflects a situation in your waking life in which you are much closer to bringing your idea into the world than you previously believed. This can often happen when you make the decision to release yourself from the expectations of other people.

AWAKEN YOUR POTENTIAL

It helps to have an objective and flexible mindset in this scenario. Be more open to unforeseen opportunities to put your concept into practice quickly. The more open you are to opportunity, the more fortunate encounters you will have. In which situation might you release yourself from the judgement of others in order to put one of your ideas into action?

This dream is a waking-life reflection of a surprise opportunity to bring your ideas into the world and to drive your ideas forward. If, on the other hand, you feel no real ownership of the eventual outcome of all your hard work, then you might be dreaming of giving birth to the wrong baby.

Wrong baby

UNLOCK THE MEANING

A dream in which you give birth to the wrong baby indicates a situation in your waking life in which you may feel that all your efforts are being directed towards putting someone else's idea into practice. It may also suggest that someone has taken your idea but put it into practice in a way that is unworkable.

AWAKEN YOUR POTENTIAL

How might you nurture and develop one of your own ideas rather than always bringing the plans of others into fruition? Think about how you might steer and contribute to the development to set it back on track: you will enjoy more rewarding results. Instead of disowning all your hard work, realize that you now have the experience and skill to put one of your own ideas into practice.

_____

Another dream about a baby's birth is that of an unusual baby who might not even materialize in human form.

Unusual baby

UNLOCK THE MEANING

Dreaming of giving birth to an unusual baby often signifies that the practical implementation of your idea didn't turn out as you initially expected. This baby might not be a baby at all but an object or an animal or even an alien. Even though your labour of love doesn't live up to your idealized expectations, you have still created a practical outcome that you can continue to develop.

AWAKEN YOUR POTENTIAL

Work with what you have created to bring it closer to the result that you originally conceived. The practical side of bringing other aspects to life may take longer than you thought. Challenge yourself to make the most out of this situation, even if it isn't the outcome you had first expected.

Death Dreams

Dreaming of death can be unsettling, but dreams about dying are rarely about an actual death in your waking life. When you create a dream that involves a death, you are becoming more aware of a fundamental transformation in your waking life. This transformation often involves moving on from a situation that you no longer find fulfilling. By respectfully laying the past to rest, you give yourself the opportunity to step into a better future. Rather than feeling that you always have to live in the past, dreams of death allow you to honour past achievements so you can move forward.

Own death

UNLOCK THE MEANING

Dreaming of your own death does not mean that your life is in any danger of ending. Instead, it indicates an opportunity to transform some of your habitual behaviours so that you can step fully into a new future by naturally letting go of aspects of your past.

AWAKEN YOUR POTENTIAL

Think about some of your habitual behaviours and decide whether they are helping you move forward or are holding you back. Be open to stepping outside your comfort zone and letting go of what no longer works for you. Can you transform some of your behavioural patterns to step fully into a new opportunity?

This unnerving dream can prove disturbing for the dreamer, but it can be even more unsettling to dream of the death of a loved one. Again, this is not a premonition. Instead, it is an invitation to channel one of your characteristic behaviours in a new way.

Loved one's death

UNLOCK THE MEANING

When you dream of a loved one, you are using them to symbolize the characteristic quality that you associate with them. Dreaming of their death reflects a waking-life situation in which you have the opportunity to transform how you use that characteristic quality yourself.

AWAKEN YOUR POTENTIAL

Give yourself the freedom to behave in different ways and embody those qualities you associate with your loved one. For example, you may routinely rely on your loved one to show compassion because you feel you might appear weak to others if you showed yourself to be compassionate. By opening up to the possibility of displaying compassion yourself, you no longer have to rely on others to be compassionate for you, as you may have done in the past. What one quality do you associate most with the loved one in your dream and how can you embody that quality yourself in waking life?

Whereas dreaming of a loved one's death reflects the need to let go of a reliance on others to display particular qualities, a dead person returning indicates the opportunity to embody and express behaviours you associated with that person.

Dead person returns

UNLOCK THE MEANING

It may be that your loved one has passed away in waking life, but they appear in your dream as large as life and seemingly still alive. Dreaming of a dead person returning from beyond the grave symbolizes an opportunity for you to recreate some of their personal qualities and to reconnect a part of your identity that you felt you had lost forever.

AWAKEN YOUR POTENTIAL

Embrace and embody the qualities that you admired the most in your loved one. Consider how might you express this through an action you take in day-to-day life. By embodying those qualities, your loved one will continue to live on inside you.

While dreaming of deceased people is associated with their characteristic behaviours, dreaming of graves and funerals links to your current situation.

Graves and funerals

UNLOCK THE MEANING

When you dream, a grave symbolizes a situation in which you can prepare the ground for a major transformation of your current situation. A funeral represents your opportunity to acknowledge a once vital aspect of your past, so that you can peacefully lay it to rest, finding closure before moving forward.

AWAKEN YOUR POTENTIAL

What aspects of your past do you need to respectfully lay to rest so that you can move on in life? Take the time to acknowledge the aspects of your past that are no longer a vital part of your current situation. We need to acknowledge the importance of what we can achieve in the future as well as to honour what we have achieved in the past. It can be tempting to dwell in the past and rest on our laurels, but that can limit our freedom to explore new opportunities for personal growth.

While official burial ceremonies symbolize the process of respectfully moving on from past achievements, burying a body without official permission in a dream is often about reviving something of significance to you rather than releasing yourself from it.

Disposing of a body

UNLOCK THE MEANING

Dreaming that you are trying to dispose of a body by some unofficial method can indicate that you are trying to bring some aspect of yourself into life rather than finally laying it to rest. Disposing of a body in a dream symbolizes that you feel that circumstances may have forced you to conceal some essential aspect of yourself in waking life. This may be a particular creative talent that you feel you had to abandon to meet the expectations of other people.

AWAKEN YOUR POTENTIAL

Realize that you have an opportunity to resurrect a neglected talent and choose whether you want to reveal it to other people or conceal it so you will be accepted by them. In which situation might you be in grave danger of abandoning an activity that would make your life more fulfilling?

If, contrastingly, you dream that you are accountable for the death of the person, it indicates that you feel personally responsible for abandoning your creative talent.

Guilty of murder

UNLOCK THE MEANING

When you dream of being guilty of murder, this represents a waking-life situation in which you are actively trying to eliminate some creative aspect of your character. This aspect seems to be at odds with how you currently see yourself and appears to be incompatible with your idealized self-image.

AWAKEN YOUR POTENTIAL

What creative aspects of your character might you be trying to eliminate because they don't seem to fit in with the self-image you want to project? Rather than trying to conform to this sense of who you are, give yourself the authority to behave more naturally so that you can have the freedom to find out who you really are deep down.

If you dream of large-scale death and destruction, rather than just the deaths of individuals, then this suggests a major transformation in your day-to-day life.

End of the world

UNLOCK THE MEANING

Dreams with apocalyptic events, such as earthquakes or asteroid strikes, symbolize a situation in which you have a great opportunity to transform your waking life completely. The upheaval may seem unwelcome, but it gives you the chance to eliminate hidden stresses that have been bubbling away underneath the surface.

AWAKEN YOUR POTENTIAL

Instead of thinking that this is the end of everything, see the upheaval as an opportunity to leave behind aspects of your life that no longer bring you any value or satisfaction. Ask yourself how you might completely transform a situation by stepping into your power.

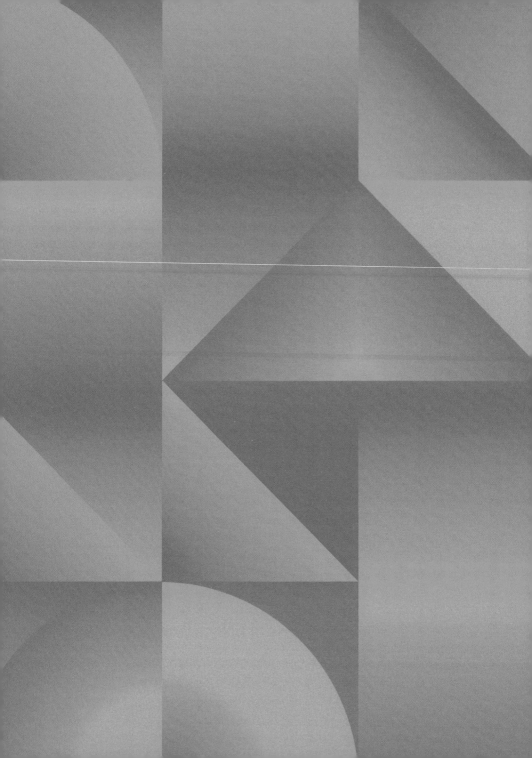

WORK & PLAY

When we are at work, we may think that we have to hide our emotions and not reveal how we really feel about situations. Although this may help us to maintain a professional image during the day, we naturally process our concealed emotions in our dreams at night. We use work situations in our dreams to symbolize how we value and assess our talents in our actual working lives. We also use playing situations in dreams to experiment with how we can creatively use our talents to achieve our goals in waking life.

In this chapter, you will find out the significance of how you identify your deeper purpose in different dream scenarios: why work dreams are not really about work, how confidence is connected to performing, the difference between work and play dreams and what your dream job can reveal about your true purpose in life. To take your work and play dream work further, try the exercise on page 171.

Work Dreams

When you dream of work colleagues and workplace situations, you are using them to explore your fundamental values and how you express these to the people around you. In waking life, organizations often use annual reviews to assess employee performance and give feedback. When you dream, you provide yourself with a nightly assessment of how valued you feel by others and, more importantly, how much you value yourself. You use your work colleagues to symbolize characteristic qualities that you consider to be valuable. Dream workplace situations are used to represent waking-life situations in which you have the opportunity to express your value.

Catching a train

UNLOCK THE MEANING

Catching a train in a dream symbolizes embarking on a particular path of professional progression. This will lead to a predetermined outcome within a known time frame. Although this provides a sense of steady and certain progress, it can also limit your freedom to explore other opportunities and this may cause you to hesitate.

AWAKEN YOUR POTENTIAL

Commit yourself to following a known professional path for a specific amount of time. After this, use this juncture to pause and review whether this is the path you want to stay on. Trying to keep your options open might mean you miss an opportunity to get ahead, so calculate the risks involved in being noncommittal against the potential of the career trajectory you are on.

The feeling of having limited professional opportunities is also experienced in dreaming of being trapped in a lift.

Trapped in a lift

UNLOCK THE MEANING

Dreaming of being trapped in a lift can often reflect your frustrations about working through the various levels of your professional development. You may feel stuck in your promotion prospects and unable to open the doors to new opportunities.

AWAKEN YOUR POTENTIAL

Start thinking outside the box about alternative professional development pathways. What other routes might you explore? See what other steps you can take, even if it requires a bit of effort. Think about other ways to achieve the professional levels you aspire to, such as moving to a higher position in a different organization or starting your own business and building it from the ground up.

The response to being trapped in a lift, both in your dreams and in waking life, is to push the lift buttons in the hope that you can get the lift moving again or communicate with someone who can help you. Pushing the wrong button or dialling the wrong number also features widely in work dreams.

Wrong number or button

UNLOCK THE MEANING

When you dream that you keep pressing the wrong button or dialling the wrong number, it indicates a waking-life situation in which you find it challenging to communicate with a particular person. This is often because you are focused on getting your message across to them and not paying enough attention to understanding how they are responding to you.

AWAKEN YOUR POTENTIAL

Rather than persistently trying to push your ideas on to another person, be more open to what they are trying to say to you. Make it a conversation. How might you change your communication style so that you can clearly express your needs to the people around you?

We are used to experiencing a simple cause-and-effect process when we push a button or dial a number. That is why we feel so frustrated when this method goes awry. We tend to have similar expectations of the technology that we use, trusting that it will always respond in a reliable manner.

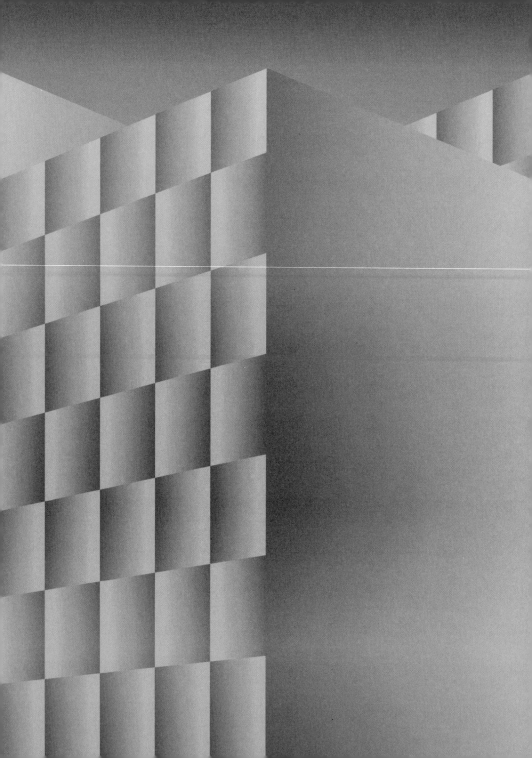

Malfunctioning technology

UNLOCK THE MEANING

Dreaming of malfunctioning technology usually symbolizes a waking-life situation in which there has been a breakdown in communication with someone you habitually rely on. This can often be a result of taking that person for granted and not appreciating what they need from you by way of support.

AWAKEN YOUR POTENTIAL

Maintain the quality of your connections with other people by being attentive to their needs as well as your own; don't wait to fix relationships until after they have broken down, but take pre-emptive action. Checking in and nurturing your connections is the best way of avoiding communication breakdowns and improving the health and benefits of your relationships.

As well as communicating directly through our speech, we also communicate indirectly through body language and our clothing. The clothes (or lack of clothes) that we wear in a dream symbolize the self-image we wish to present to others.

Naked in public

UNLOCK THE MEANING

Being naked in public in a dream reflects circumstances in waking life in which you feel exposed and vulnerable to the judgement and potential criticism of others. This can often occur when you find yourself in an unfamiliar professional situation and are unsure of the most appropriate way to present yourself.

AWAKEN YOUR POTENTIAL

It may seem more comfortable to try and conceal your vulnerability by presenting an inauthentic self-image. However, the more you are able to reveal your authentic self, the more that other people are likely to trust and open up to you. Consider the occasions when you can be more open about displaying your knowledge and experience to others.

It can be challenging to open up to the people whom you work with, particularly those who may be in senior positions to you. If you feel you have spoken out of turn or are not toeing the company line, this might be imagined in a dream as being fired.

Being fired

UNLOCK THE MEANING

Dreaming of being fired does not mean you are about to be dismissed. Being fired in a dream symbolizes that you are getting fired up about employing your skills and experience to support a deeper purpose. It can be easy to become too comfortable in a job that you have outgrown and dreaming of being fired suggests that a new opportunity is sparking your ambition.

AWAKEN YOUR POTENTIAL

How might you employ your skills and experience to support your deeper purpose in life? Take some time to consider what that purpose might be, and look for opportunities to use your talents to help you fulfil it.

In dreams, work symbolizes your deeper purpose in life and workplaces represent situations in which you can valuably employ that purpose.

Empty workplace

UNLOCK THE MEANING

Dreaming that you are in an empty workplace can indicate that your professional talents are not being fully acknowledged and valued by other people in your waking life. This can often happen when you move from one type of job to another and you have yet to fully demonstrate your abilities to your new colleagues. It can also occur if your working routine has significantly changed and you feel you are not yet able to show your skills to their fullest extent.

AWAKEN YOUR POTENTIAL

Rather than waiting for your abilities to be recognized and appreciated by other people, take pride in your knowledge and skills. The more purposeful you are in the work that you do, the more you will be valued by others. Working with purpose enables you to focus your efforts and consistently produce valuable results, rather than just appearing busy and actually producing very little in the process.

Play Dreams

Work and play can seem to be quite distinct activities, but they are closely connected in your dreams. When you dream about work, you are considering your value to others and to yourself. When you dream about play, you are reflecting on how well you are performing in waking life and actively displaying your abilities to others. When you consider your performance in day-to-day life, you are not just thinking about your involvement in creative or sporting activities, but in any situation in which you can confidently display your unique skills to others and have them appreciated by a wider audience.

Public performance

UNLOCK THE MEANING

Dreaming of performing in public signifies a situation in your waking life in which you have the opportunity to recognize your own talents. You may find it challenging to display your talents in the dream, reflecting a tendency towards being critical of your abilities in waking life.

AWAKEN YOUR POTENTIAL

Recognize and accept your talent rather than always judging it harshly. The more comfortable you are with your abilities, the more likely you are to be able to improve them. Stop looking to others for approval and take confidence in your known strengths.

Dreaming of a public performance can involve a realization that you are using the wrong equipment. For example, you may be using a pool cue to play golf or an electric guitar to play tennis.

Wrong equipment

UNLOCK THE MEANING

Dreaming of having the wrong equipment for the particular sport or performance that you are involved in often indicates that you feel unable to apply your skills in a waking-life situation. This is usually because you are being overly rigid in your approach rather than adapting your skills to the current challenge.

AWAKEN YOUR POTENTIAL

Be more open to experimenting with your talents and experiences so that you can apply them in different ways. Adapting your skill-set to new challenges can open up many more opportunities for you. How might you adapt one of your skills so that you can succeed with a current challenge?

Feeling that you have to use your talents in a very particular manner can also be reflected in dreams in which you are engaged in a tense battle with an invincible opponent.

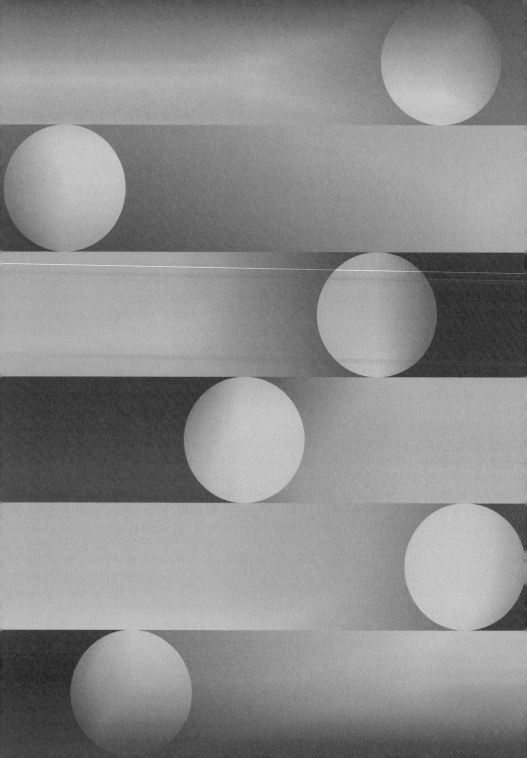

Unbeatable opponent

UNLOCK THE MEANING

The unbeatable opponent in your dream symbolizes some aspect of yourself that you feel is weak and vulnerable. You fear that this vulnerability might be exploited by other people. You feel that you have to fight endlessly with this weakness so that you appear strong and indestructible to others. You can win the battle by accepting your vulnerabilities.

AWAKEN YOUR POTENTIAL

Accept those aspects of yourself that you feel may be weak and flawed. The best performers are those who work on their weaknesses rather than just display their strengths. How might you work on developing your perceived weaknesses rather than simply trying to cover them up?

If you are in a situation in your waking life in which you feel weak or lack confidence, you may dream that you are involved in some never-ending game.

Never-ending game

UNLOCK THE MEANING

Dreaming of participating in a never-ending game indicates a waking-life situation in which you are continually playing around with idealized outcomes. The game – sometimes a sporting fixture or an immersive computer game – seems never-ending because you may lack the confidence to commit to taking the actions necessary to ensure a practical outcome.

AWAKEN YOUR POTENTIAL

Rather than playing around with your options, commit yourself to taking decisive action and clearly identify what would be an acceptable result for you. Think about one decision you can make right now that will offer a realistic outcome.

Play is often considered to be a physical or creative activity. At a deeper level, however, play is fundamentally an emotional experience. For example, a swimming dream reflects a waking-life opportunity to immerse yourself in emotional exploration.

Swimming pool

UNLOCK THE MEANING

Water in dreams symbolizes feelings and emotions. A swimming pool represents a waking-life situation in which you feel that you have to contain your emotions as you play around to achieve a favourable result. This can result in you feeling unable to apply the real depth of your knowledge and experience.

AWAKEN YOUR POTENTIAL

Be open to sharing your deeper emotions about a situation you are involved with. Letting your feelings flow can be self-motivating and energizing. In which circumstances do you feel that you are suppressing deep emotions that need to be expressed?

As you engage with waking-life challenges and play around with possible outcomes, your dreams of play can often involve limitations, such as unbeatable opponents, never-ending games and emotional constraints. As you resolve these challenges in waking life, you may dream of running free.

Running free

UNLOCK THE MEANING

In dreams, running symbolizes an ability to motivate yourself so that you can quickly take some powerful steps to facilitate a chosen outcome. Running free in a dream indicates a waking-life situation in which you have taken steps to move beyond any limitations that may have been imposed upon you; you feel liberated in your pursuit of a personal ambition.

AWAKEN YOUR POTENTIAL

Direct your energy into your current challenge. What will get you really motivated about the result that you want to arrive at? Identify any hurdles and obstacles in your way and take the steps you need to overcome them. How can you use your energy and self-motivation to move beyond a situation that may have been holding you back?

While running free signifies overcoming limitations placed in your path, when you dream of winning at sport, you are considering the limitations you may be placing on yourself and how you can conquer these fears and doubts.

Winning at sport

UNLOCK THE MEANING

Winning at an individual sport in a dream may involve competing against someone else, but it means that you are actually competing against your own performance and raising your game. Winning in a team sport suggests that you are successfully attracting the assistance of others to help you achieve your ambitions.

AWAKEN YOUR POTENTIAL

Conquer your fears and doubts by acknowledging them and actively engaging with them. This will give you the opportunity to achieve your ambitions. In any performance in waking life, your most skilled opponent will always be that self-critical voice in your head.

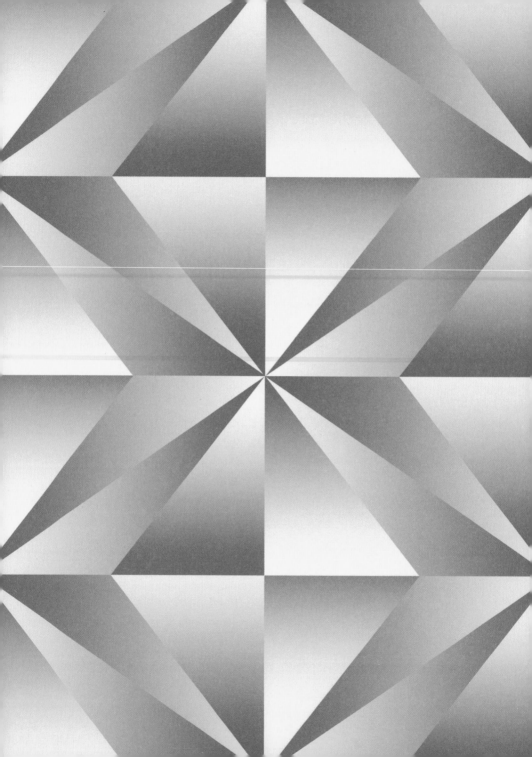

WEALTH
& HEALTH

Many of us daydream about having financial wealth in waking life and the feelings of power and choice that this can provide. Our night-time dreams of wealth use symbols of financial abundance to help us explore and access the wealth of self-knowledge that we have accumulated. Although that inner wealth may appear to have no financial value, richness of experience is one of the most valuable things we can possess. That wealth of self-knowledge also emerges in our dreams about waking-life health situations, which we can use to develop and maintain a healthy sense of well-being.

In this chapter, you will discover the significance of how you develop your knowledge and experience in different dream scenarios: why health dreams are not about being unhealthy, how stress is connected to health dreams, the difference between wealth and health dreams and why your wealth of experience can be one of your most valuable assets. To take your wealth and health dream work further, try the exercise on page 172.

Wealth Dreams

Wealth dreams represent situations in your waking life in which you are reflecting on the accumulated value of your work and performances. It can be tempting to think that wealth is just a tangible value, which you accumulate through good fortune and lose through bad fortune. Rather than simply trying to add up the value of your material assets, however, your wealth dreams are enabling you to understand the greater value of human qualities – those that often seem intangible. By developing those intangible human qualities, you often generate opportunities to develop your inner wealth. The more that you do this, the more fortunate you can become.

Bank robbery

UNLOCK THE MEANING

A bank in a dream symbolizes the valuable wealth of experience and knowledge that you are accumulating throughout your life. Being involved in a bank robbery indicates a waking-life situation in which you feel that other people are taking full credit for what you have produced rather than recognizing and honouring you for it.

AWAKEN YOUR POTENTIAL

Make sure that other people acknowledge the value of your experience and skills, and that they give you the credit that you richly deserve. Have the confidence and courage to claim ownership of your valuable contribution and ensure that you are credited for it. Think about occasions when other people have drawn on your expertise without recognizing the value of your contribution.

When you dream, money symbolizes how much you value yourself and how much you feel that other people value you. The dreamt loss of a valuable often links to the former.

Loss of a valuable

UNLOCK THE MEANING

Dreaming that you have lost something valuable, such as purse, wallet or jewellery, suggests that your sense of self-worth in waking life has been substantially reduced in some way. This can often happen as you transition from one period of your life to another. You may hold others accountable for your loss, but you are ultimately responsible for having your value recognized by other people.

AWAKEN YOUR POTENTIAL

Rather than helplessly waiting for other people to recognize the value of your talents and skills, learn to rectify this same flaw within yourself: learn to truly value yourself and realize that you have a lot to offer. How might you draw attention to your valuable experience so that you can make a worthwhile contribution to a situation?

We often don't value ourselves enough because we lack confidence in our resourcefulness. Even though you may not have the financial means you desire, being creatively resourceful naturally opens up opportunities for you.

No money

UNLOCK THE MEANING

If you dream of being penniless, then this indicates a waking-life situation in which you can create value by using your inner resourcefulness and wealth of knowledge. You can start to gain the recognition that you richly deserve by confidently demonstrating your talents to other people.

AWAKEN YOUR POTENTIAL

Believe in your skills and experience. They have value. Realize that you have an abundance of accumulated expertise. Do not invest in the fear that you might perform poorly. The more confidence that you have in your skills and abilities, the more often opportunities to use them will seem to emerge in your waking life.

Realizing that you have the inner resourcefulness and talent to create value will naturally attract rich rewards in waking life.

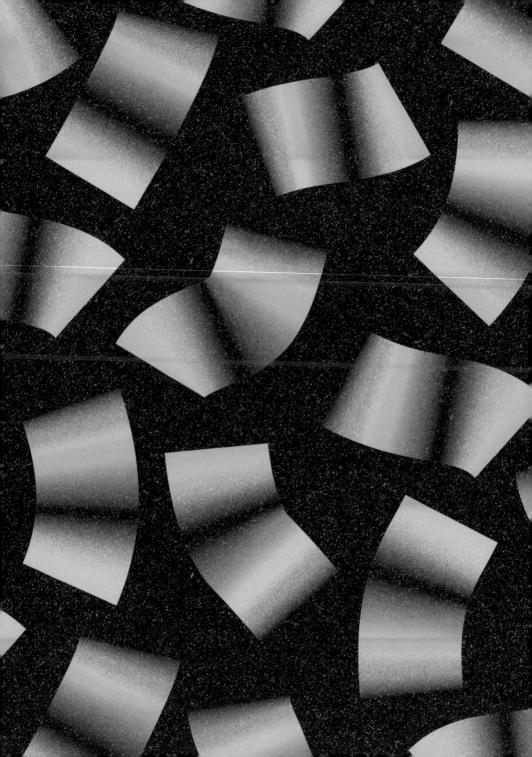

Finding money

UNLOCK THE MEANING

Finding money in a dream, perhaps just lying on the ground or in the form of cash stuffed into a large suitcase, indicates that you have been largely unaware of how creative and resourceful you can be. As you find more confidence in yourself, you will find more valuable opportunities open up in waking life.

AWAKEN YOUR POTENTIAL

When you dream of finding money somewhere obvious, it indicates that you are becoming more aware of opportunities that no one else has seen yet. Be more open in your day-to-day life to finding unconventional ways to use your talents and experience. Stepping outside your comfort zone will help you find new opportunities to create and add value.

Contrastingly, if you find buried treasure in a dream, it suggests that you may have been hiding your talents but now have an opportunity to display them.

Buried treasure

UNLOCK THE MEANING

Dreaming of buried treasure reflects a situation in your waking life in which you felt you had to conceal your creativity and resourcefulness. Although you may have been trying to protect these assets by hiding them from others, you may also have been hiding them from yourself.

AWAKEN YOUR POTENTIAL

Reveal your wealth of accumulated knowledge, talent and expertise to others and to yourself. Doing this may require that you dig deeper into your resourcefulness, but the outcome will be rewarding. Display your experience so your value can be more fully recognized.

Finding buried treasure reflects how we often view our ability to gain wealth as random good fortune rather than as a result of developing our talents. Winning a fortune on the lottery is another dream in which you seem to gain a lot of wealth very quickly through a seemingly random event.

Winning the lottery

UNLOCK THE MEANING

Dreaming of winning the lottery suggests that you have been suddenly and unexpectedly presented with a valuable opportunity in your waking life. Although it may seem that it has required little effort on your part, the reality is that your talents and expertise are rapidly becoming a winning combination.

AWAKEN YOUR POTENTIAL

Start celebrating your creative gifts and expertise. Although they might seem quite minor at the moment, the more you display them, the more that other people will be attracted to your value. Seize the moment and make your own luck: how can you use your creativity and problem-solving skills to make the most of an unexpected opportunity?

A popular ambition for lottery winners, and would-be lottery winners, is to buy a bigger house. This dream presents an opportunity for upgrading your life experience through self-development.

Buying a bigger house

UNLOCK THE MEANING

As a house symbolizes the self in a dream, buying and living in a bigger house represents opportunities for expanding your personal development in waking life. It reflects a situation in which you can use your wealth of talent and expertise to grow and flourish as an individual.

AWAKEN YOUR POTENTIAL

You may feel that your personal development is complete, but there is always room to grow. Do a personal survey of your accumulated skills and experience and consider how you might valuably develop them even further. How might you use your skills and experience in waking life to open the door to a new opportunity?

Health Dreams

When you dream of health, you are not reflecting on your physical health, or the health of others, in waking life. Instead, you are considering how healthy or unhealthy a situation in your waking life might be. Although you may try to diagnose an unhealthy situation in an objective and analytical way in waking life, your health dreams help you to understand how you really feel. Rather than being ill at ease and unable to remedy the waking-life situation, work with your dreams to discover what will make you feel better.

Toilet troubles

UNLOCK THE MEANING

A toilet symbolizes a place where you can attend to your own needs by releasing what is no longer healthy or nourishing. Having toilet troubles in your dreams suggests that you feel embarrassed about voicing your needs. This may be because you are always looking after the needs of others rather than attending to your own. Toilet dreams reflect situations in waking life in which you can feel challenged to let go of what you no longer need.

AWAKEN YOUR POTENTIAL

How can you openly ask for help from others to fulfil your personal needs instead of feeling embarrassed to do so? Bravely set some personal boundaries so that other people understand that you have to look after your needs as well as theirs.

We also use our bodily functions and parts to symbolize aspects of our life that we are keen to retain.

Teeth falling out

UNLOCK THE MEANING

Dreaming that your teeth are falling out indicates a waking-life situation in which you feel that you are losing the confidence to assert yourself. You display your teeth when you are smiling or biting, and so they symbolize how confident and self-assertive you are feeling.

AWAKEN YOUR POTENTIAL

Be more confident in whatever is currently challenging you in your waking life. You always have more power to assert yourself than you think you do. It can be tempting to put on a smile that you don't really feel in an attempt to keep other people happy, but you can often reach a more successful outcome for everyone by being assertive rather than just accepting situations that make you unhappy.

When you dream that larger parts of your body are missing, this indicates a waking-life situation in which you feel detached and unable to take action in the way you normally do.

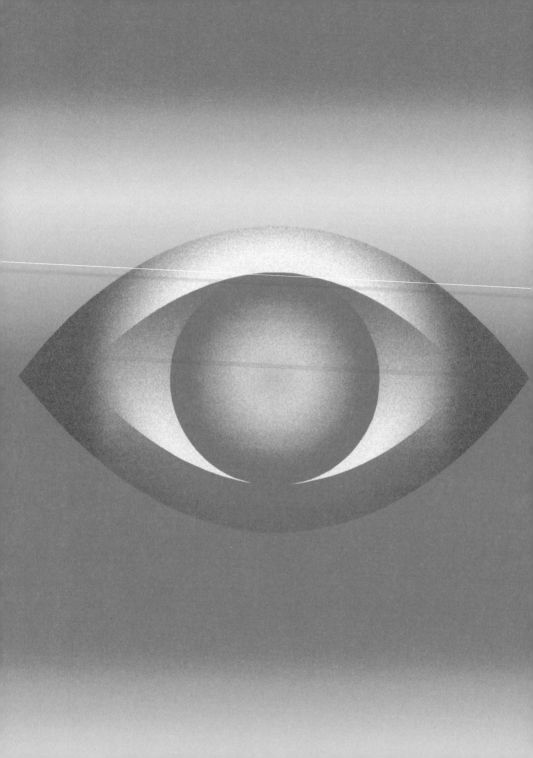

Missing body part

UNLOCK THE MEANING

Dreaming that you are missing a body part, such as your limbs or your head, suggests that you are viewing a waking-life situation in an unusually detached manner, which is caused by feelings of powerless. Although you may lack the power to do anything yourself, actively connecting with other people will help you take the vital actions that are necessary. Legs and feet symbolize your ability to take the steps you need, and arms and hands symbolize your ability to control a situation.

AWAKEN YOUR POTENTIAL

Rather than just feeling powerless, have the confidence to ask other people to lend you a hand until you can find your feet again. Connecting with other people and allowing them to support you is the best way to re-establish your sense of individual power.

Dreaming that your body is intact but that you are unable to move can reflect a day-to-day situation in which you are struggling to find the motivation you need.

Unable to move

UNLOCK THE MEANING

If you dream that you are unable to move a part of your body, this suggests a waking-life situation in which you are finding it difficult to make a decision. This can sometimes happen when you are unclear about your motives in deciding what action to take, resulting in paralysis by analysis, whereby you are focusing all your efforts on possible outcomes rather than committing yourself to action.

AWAKEN YOUR POTENTIAL

Get the situation moving by committing to at least one decision. Even a small commitment will help you move to action. When might you be overthinking potential solutions to a problem rather than taking action?

If you feel paralyzed or stuck in an emotionally unhealthy situation and feel there is no immediate or obvious remedy for it, this might appear as some form of life-threatening illness.

Life-threatening illness

UNLOCK THE MEANING

Various types of life-threatening illness in dreams represent different kinds of emotional unease in waking life. For example, cardiac conditions indicate relationships where your heart really isn't in it any more. A wasting disease suggests that you are wasting your time in an emotional relationship.

AWAKEN YOUR POTENTIAL

Take care to look after your emotional health as well as your physical health. If a situation is causing you to feel ill at ease, perhaps even chronically so, then take positive action to remedy it. In which of your relationships do you need to restore a healthy emotional balance?

In the same way that we may try to heal our physical ailments ourselves, we often try to work through our emotional tensions alone. Sometimes, however, we have to ask other people to help us – this can manifest as dreams in which professional health workers are giving us care and attention.

Hospital visit

UNLOCK THE MEANING

A hospital symbolizes a situation in waking life in which you have the opportunity to resolve emotional tensions by asking for help from other people. We often try to conceal our emotional tensions from others because we don't want to burden them with our problems. That can be very stressful and result in feelings of unease. These emotional tensions are often resolved when you open up your heart to others and realize that they really care about how you feel.

AWAKEN YOUR POTENTIAL

Rather than nursing relationship grievances and bottling up tension, have the confidence to ask other people for advice and support. Making an admission of how you really feel will provide a healthy start to the healing process.

As well as feeling unhealthy in a dream, you may feel so healthy and powerful that you appear to have superhuman powers. You might find yourself having unbelievable strength and incredible abilities, such as X-ray vision.

Superpower

UNLOCK THE MEANING

Dreams of possessing a superpower often arise when you feel powerless to escape from a waking-life situation that is making you feel ill at ease. Your superpowers, however, indicate that you have the inner resourcefulness you need to move mountains (in dreams of super strength) and see right through any questionable behaviours (as in X-ray vision).

AWAKEN YOUR POTENTIAL

Have the courage to step into your power when a person or situation is making you feel uncomfortable. Rather than waiting for others to rescue you, realize you have the power to rescue yourself. How can you use your resourcefulness to right some wrongs?

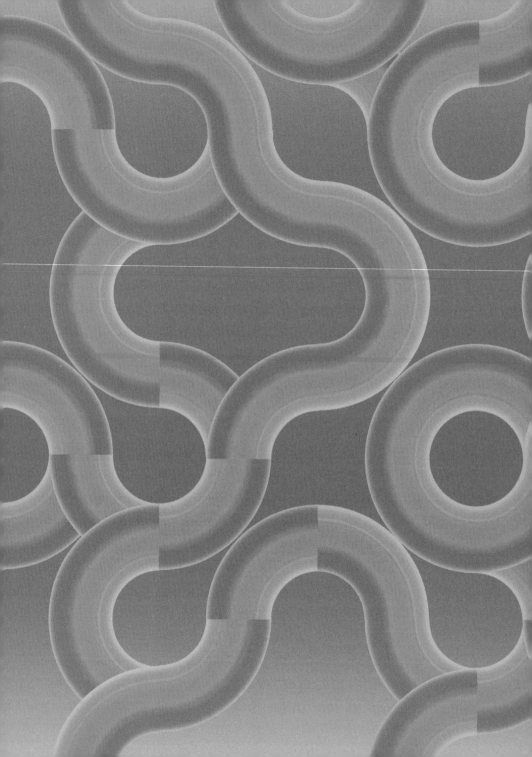

TRAVEL & DISCOVERY

Dreaming gives you the freedom to travel into your inner world and discover a wide range of different perspectives on how to make progress in your waking life. Rather than just having one fixed viewpoint, you have the opportunity to look at waking-life situations in a number of different ways. The journeys you make in your dreams are a natural process of self-exploration in which you can find out more about who you actually are, what you really need and what you truly believe. The insight you gain in your dreams naturally broadens your horizons and opens up more possibilities in your waking life.

In this chapter, you will discover the significance of different dream scenarios: why travel dreams are about inner journeys, how discovery dreams are connected to your future self, the difference between travel and discovery dreams and how your dream discoveries can help you find chances to develop in waking life. To take your travel and discovery dream work further, try the exercise on page 172.

Travel
Dreams

When you travel in the outer world in your waking life, you may
set out on a journey with a particular destination in mind or you
may just find yourself wandering and seeing where you end up.
The same processes happen in your inner world when you dream.
You may use your dreams to reach a particular understanding of a
specific waking-life situation. You also may find yourself wandering
(and wondering) to see what new perspectives might emerge.
Your travel dreams also reflect your waking-life ambitions and how
much progress you feel you are making towards them.

Taking the wrong route

UNLOCK THE MEANING

Dreaming of taking the wrong route signifies that you are not following the path that you would like to in your waking life. Even though you feel that you may be stuck in a rut, it might seem that changing direction is too risky and so it is safer just to stick with your current route.

AWAKEN YOUR POTENTIAL

Take some time and consider what you really want to achieve in your life. Changing direction may seem hazardous but so is always trying to play it safe and never feeling fulfilled. How might you make some small changes in your life that will help you start to head in the direction that is most motivating for you?

At other times in your dreams, you know the path you want to take, but it feels like you just cannot maintain your chosen course of action. This might appear in your dream as a car spinning out of control.

Out-of-control vehicle

UNLOCK THE MEANING

Any time you create a dream involving a vehicle, you are considering how you can make progress towards a desired outcome in your waking life. Being in an out-of-control vehicle suggests that you feel you are losing command of your ability to make progress towards your chosen goal.

AWAKEN YOUR POTENTIAL

Rather than panicking at your fear that you've lost all control of a situation, guide it back on course by asking for help from others as you drive forward with your ambitions. In which situation might you be driving yourself too hard but assistance could be available?

One of the overriding concerns in an out-of-control vehicle dream is that you will be involved in a crash or fall into a dangerous situation. Falling seems to be the ultimate loss of control, resulting in complete failure to achieve your chosen outcome.

Free falling

UNLOCK THE MEANING

Falling is often associated with failure in waking life, but in a dream, falling symbolizes your opportunity to relax your grip on a situation in which you are trying to exert too much control. As you release control, your desired outcome will often naturally fall into place.

AWAKEN YOUR POTENTIAL

Rather than clinging to your need to control everything and attempting to micromanage all possible outcomes, try guiding and influencing instead. How can you exert a positive influence on a situation you previously held too closely to your chest, or consider whether you should simply step back and allow things to take shape?

When you are in a waking-life situation in which there are a number of people involved in some form of collective failure, your dreams may feature an aircraft crash.

Aircraft crash

UNLOCK THE MEANING

In dreams, the sky symbolizes your thought processes and ideas, and since aircraft are vehicles of the skies, they represent your ability to get an idea off the ground and then to land it in practical reality. A dreamed aircraft crash represents a situation in your waking life in which you may need to use a more down-to-earth approach to complete a complex project successfully.

AWAKEN YOUR POTENTIAL

If a complex plan appears to be falling apart, have the confidence to take decisive control and practical steps to achieve your chosen outcome. Although it may seem easier to stay in the realm of theories, at some point you will have to put your ideas into practice. How might you take a more practical approach and overcome your idealization of the potential outcomes?

While aircrafts symbolize plans and ideas that you are setting in motion and hoping to complete successfully, missing a plane suggests you feel you are missing opportunities.

Missing a plane

UNLOCK THE MEANING

When you dream of missing a plane, this suggests that you are working to a tight schedule in waking life but won't be able to meet the timetable you have set yourself. This is often because you are spending lots of your time charting out your plans without actually managing to put them into action.

AWAKEN YOUR POTENTIAL

Get your plan moving. Even though it may feel that you don't have all the details to be sure of a certain outcome yet, the alternative is to fail to complete your mission. In which situation can you take specific and purposeful action to achieve a personal ambition rather than just keeping yourself busy?

_____

You may be in the process of gathering all the resources you think you need to put your plans into action so that you can deal with any eventuality. This continuous preparation might appear as a packing dream.

Endless packing

UNLOCK THE MEANING

When you find yourself endlessly packing in a dream, it suggests that you think your plan will succeed simply by possessing all the resources you need. This often results in an endless acquisition of resources to prepare for every eventuality rather than committing yourself to a particular course of action.

AWAKEN YOUR POTENTIAL

Take action and begin your journey with the resources you currently have. Trust that you have the inner resourcefulness you need and that you have accumulated enough expertise already. Trying to prepare for every eventuality can weigh you down and can also burden you with obligations and commitments that prevent progress.

When you finally commit to action in waking life, you can often experience a sense of release and freedom, and this might appear in a dream in which you can fly.

Flying

UNLOCK THE MEANING

Dreaming of flying indicates that you have liberated yourself from some weighty limitation that has been holding you back in waking life. This often occurs when you use your creativity and problem-solving skills to rise above a major challenge you have been facing, and so you can now make much speedier progress.

AWAKEN YOUR POTENTIAL

Rather than just thinking up ideas to solve a problem, try putting some of your ideas into action, which will help you see the bigger picture and raise your overall awareness. Instead of weighing yourself down with burdensome issues that are not really your responsibility, liberate yourself from them by rising to the challenge of exploring new possibilities for personal development in your waking life.

Discovery Dreams

As you travel in your dreams, you may often find yourself in familiar and recurring locations. You may also find yourself in new and unfamiliar areas of your inner world. Dreaming is a continual process of self-discovery, and as you explore these new situations in your dreams, you are naturally exploring more about yourself. The more that you find out about yourself, the more likely you are to find the sense of fulfilment and achievement you are searching for in your waking life.

Distant lands

UNLOCK THE MEANING

When you dream of being in a distant land, this suggests that you have a waking-life opportunity to achieve something that you thought was only remotely possible. This dream can also indicate that you are exploring aspects of a waking-life situation that might seem quite foreign to you.

AWAKEN YOUR POTENTIAL

Although you may have to venture into some unfamiliar areas of thinking, you can use novel approaches to bring your success much closer. Be open to exploring different ways of understanding a challenging situation even though you don't initially feel at home with them. How might you broaden your understanding of a situation without using ideas that seem too far-fetched?

_____

You may also dream of being in a location that looks vaguely familiar, but the buildings and roads are not in the locations that you would normally expect.

Unfamiliar city or street

UNLOCK THE MEANING

Houses, and buildings in general, represent the self. When you dream of unfamiliar arrangements of buildings in cities or streets, you are thinking of the different ways you might constructively relate to an unfamiliar situation in waking life.

AWAKEN YOUR POTENTIAL

Although the outcome might seem fixed, you can create the result you want to see. Build your confidence in an unfamiliar situation by exploring a range of different perspectives so you can understand how they all connect to one another. How might you move beyond your comfort zone so that you can expand your horizons?

When you dream, the locations you visit symbolize particular situations in your waking life. Although the city or street may be unfamiliar to you in your waking life, you may find yourself returning to it again and again in your dreams.

Recurring location

UNLOCK THE MEANING

If you have recurring visits to a dream location, then you are repeatedly encountering a particular waking-life situation. If you enjoy exploring your recurring dream location, then it suggests that you are happy to continue encountering that particular waking-life situation. If you would rather not return to that dream location, then it indicates that you have the opportunity to move on from the current situation in your waking life.

AWAKEN YOUR POTENTIAL

Make the choice and decide whether you want to keep revisiting that same situation in your waking life. If not, take the first step to move on from it. It can be challenging to leave a situation that has become habitual and familiar, so ask yourself what it might take for you to step out of the comfort zone of one of your familiar habits that no longer has value for you in the way that it once did.

As you take action to move beyond a particular set of circumstances that may have been limiting opportunities for you, it can seem as if you are voyaging on a journey without apparent end, in an endless quest to an as-yet-unknown destination.

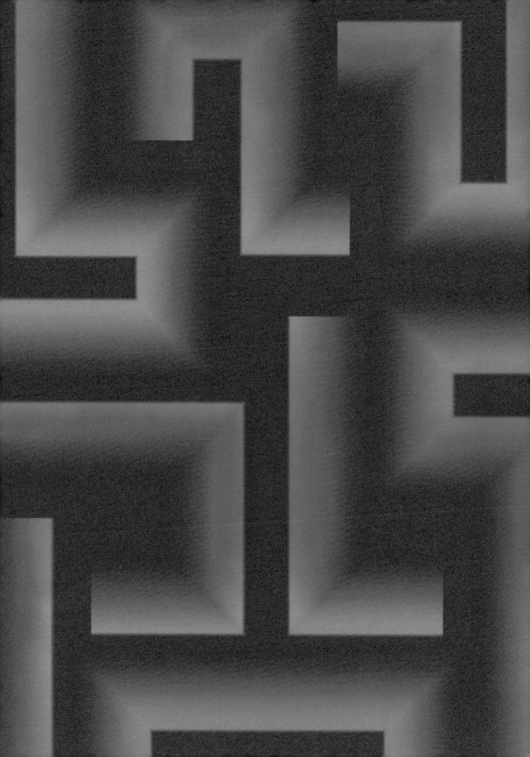

Endless quest

UNLOCK THE MEANING

Our words 'quest' and 'question' are very closely linked and dreaming of being on an endless quest suggests that your dreams are answering questions that you may not consciously be aware you are asking. The destination you are trying to reach in your dreams reflects what will bring you fulfilment in waking life.

AWAKEN YOUR POTENTIAL

Ask yourself what you truly want from your life and how you will know that you have successfully arrived at that outcome. How can you increase your awareness of a situation by exploring it further so that you can arrive at the outcome you need?

_____

As you travel on journeys of discovery in your dreams and explore where you want to go in life, you can often find yourself searching for something.

Searching for something

UNLOCK THE MEANING

Dreaming of searching for something can indicate that you are trying to discover a deeper sense of fulfilment in your day-to-day life. Although you may be trying to find it in the outer world, that deeper sense of fulfilment is invariably located in your inner world.

AWAKEN YOUR POTENTIAL

Rather than constantly searching for fulfilment in the outer world, take time to reflect on those occasions when you have found that fulfilment in your inner world. It may have been mastering a new skill that you always wanted to acquire or the successful completion of a challenge where you initially felt a bit lost. That knowledge and experience is no longer something beyond you but now successfully resides in your inner world. What is the one thing that will really bring a deep sense of fulfilment to your life?

Your search might take place outside in distant lands and unfamiliar locations, but often it takes place inside a house. A house symbolizes who you are; in discovery dreams, the house you're searching through may appear to be haunted.

Haunted house

UNLOCK THE MEANING

When you dream of being in a haunted house, you are reminding yourself of some valuable talent or personal characteristic that you have the chance to rediscover. You may have explored this talent in the past but felt that you had no real opportunity to bring it to life.

AWAKEN YOUR POTENTIAL

Give yourself the opportunity to breathe new life into a talent that you had dismissed as being of no substance in your waking life. Consider talents or personal characteristics from your past that you feel you have abandoned. Although you may have tried to close the door on them and move on, these ghosts of possibility keep coming back to haunt you with thoughts of what might have been. It may seem a little scary to revive these talents from your past, but breathing new life into them will naturally lift your spirits.

A house represents your identity, and the rooms in a house symbolize different aspects of your identity. Coming across unused rooms in your dreams indicates that you are discovering new dimensions to your identity.

Unused room

UNLOCK THE MEANING

Dreaming of an unused room often occurs when a new opportunity presents itself in your waking life. Although you may feel you know yourself very well, an unused room indicates you have talents and potential that you have yet to discover.

AWAKEN YOUR POTENTIAL

Be more open to unexpected opportunities for discovering and developing valuable personal characteristics and individual talents. It may seem easier to stay in your comfort zone, but recognizing and opening yourself up to new experiences offer you more room to expand your skills. What new possibilites to develop your potential talents and skills are you currently becoming more aware of?

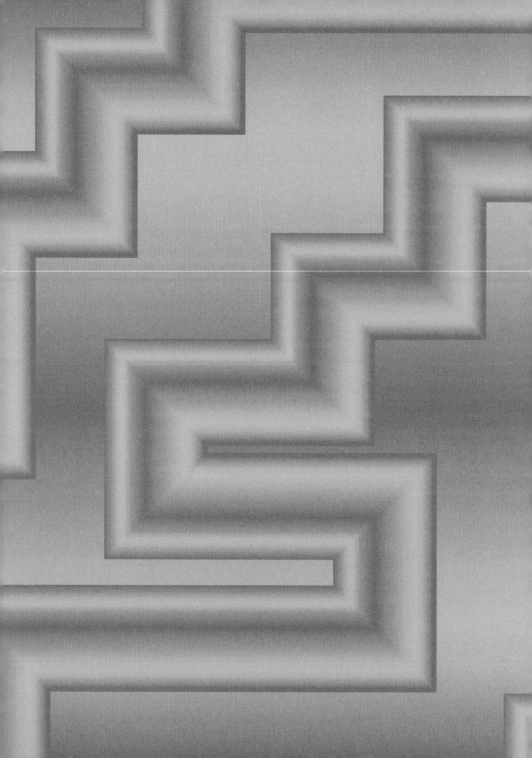

PURPOSE
& POTENTIAL

One of the most powerful ways to understand your life purpose is through working with your dreams. Your life purpose is the continual progression you make to fulfil your deepest needs in your waking life. More of these unspoken needs will emerge in your dreams as you take steps to meet them. By connecting with your life purpose in your waking life, you also connect to your wider and deeper potential.

In this chapter, you will discover how to find your real purpose in life in different dream scenarios: why purpose dreams are about committing to progress, how potential is connected to your future self, the difference between purpose and potential dreams and how potential opening up in your dreams signals new opportunity in your waking life. To take your purpose and potential dream work further, try the exercise on page 173.

Purpose Dreams

In your day-to-day life, you may sometimes question why you are doing something but you rarely give yourself the conscious opportunity to question your deeper life purpose. Your dreams provide you with the opportunity to answer those bigger questions, and explore what you find most meaningful. Purpose dreams reflect the challenges that you may encounter as you progress towards a successful outcome in your waking life. Like any worthwhile motivation in waking life, purpose dreams often involve challenges and obstacles that need to be overcome to reach a greater sense of fulfilment.

Insurmountable obstacle

UNLOCK THE MEANING

Trying to move beyond an insurmountable obstacle in a dream often indicates that you feel frustrated in your attempts to make headway in your waking life. Although the obstacle appears to be a physical object in your dream, it often represents a way in which you are holding back from achieving your waking-life purpose.

AWAKEN YOUR POTENTIAL

Rather than feeling that all barriers to your progress are external, consider the personal habits and behaviours that you can change to move forward. The insurmountable obstacle that you encounter is currently the biggest challenge in your waking life and the one you keep coming up against time after time. Big challenges often require big changes in how you deal with them. What is the biggest change you can make in your current situation?

In other dreams, it may appear that the way ahead is clear, but for some reason, you just can't take a step to make your way forward and continue with your purpose.

Can't take a step

UNLOCK THE MEANING

Your feet and legs symbolize your ability to motivate yourself and take the steps needed to make progress in a particular direction. Dreaming that you are unable to take a step can indicate that you are finding it challenging to make a first step in waking life. This first step is usually devoting yourself to a particular course of action to achieve a desired outcome. Although you are keen to reach your objective, you may be finding it difficult to make that initial commitment.

AWAKEN YOUR POTENTIAL

Self-motivation and energy are needed to face your current challenge. Commit to taking that first decisive step forward. The first step always seems the hardest, but it is the critical one that gets you moving with purpose. Each subsequent step becomes easier in turn as you find your momentum.

Even though you are keen to make that first step, you may sometimes feel unprepared and ill-equipped to commit to it. This is often reflected in dreams in which you seem to have lost your shoes or are wearing the wrong footwear.

Lost shoes

UNLOCK THE MEANING

Shoes in dreams symbolize your ability to stand up for your purpose and put it into action. Your purpose, like your shoes, has to be the right fit for you. Otherwise, you will feel uncomfortable pursuing it. Losing your shoes suggests you are becoming distracted from your purpose in waking life.

AWAKEN YOUR POTENTIAL

Have the confidence to stand up for your cause. Commit to making continued progress by minimizing distractions such as the opinions of others. Although this may seem a little uncomfortable to begin with, it is an opportunity to stand up for yourself and what you believe in, rather than being misdirected by others. Giving yourself this sense of perspective also offers you the opportunity to think about why other people hold their particular opinions and what it would be like to be standing in their shoes. Knowing where other people stand on a particular issue enables you to see the bigger picture, so you can make faster and more effective progress in your chosen purpose.

Although you may feel comfortable in the steps you are taking in the continued pursuit of your purpose, it can often seem like you are having to expend more and more effort in doing so.

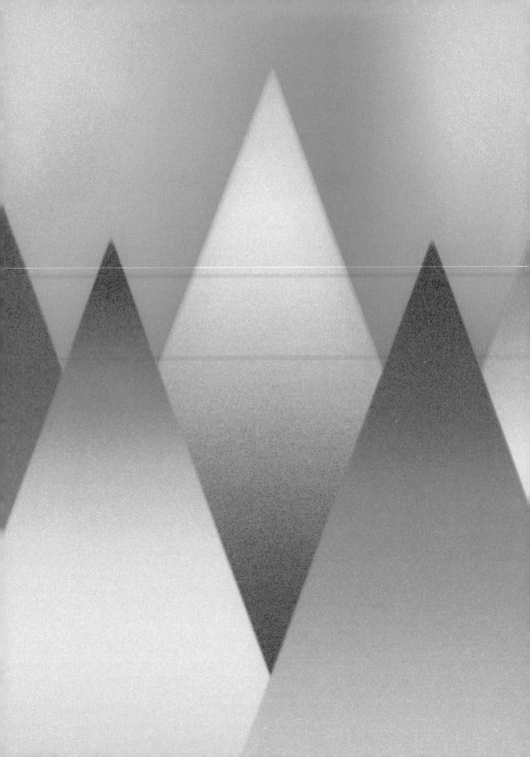

Mountain to climb

UNLOCK THE MEANING

Dreaming of climbing a mountain reflects a situation in your waking life in which you are making a sustained effort to reach a higher level of achievement. You may find that the mountainside becomes a sheer cliff in your dream, as you realize the sheer hard work that your ambition requires.

AWAKEN YOUR POTENTIAL

Prepare yourself for the long haul: progress at a steady pace rather than expending your energy in an all-out effort. Slow and steady wins the race. Ask yourself: in which situation do I need to take a more strategic, step-by-step approach to achieving my ambition?

As you purposefully continue your journey towards the outcome you desire in waking life, you will encounter apparent barriers to your progress. As well as obstacles like mountains, you may also find yourself confronting situations that seem more fluid and less certain.

Crossing a river

UNLOCK THE MEANING

Water in dreams represents your emotions and feelings. Dreaming of trying to cross a river indicates that you are facing an emotional challenge, rather than a physical challenge, as you pursue your purpose. You may feel concerned about engaging with this challenge because you fear becoming emotionally overwhelmed by it.

AWAKEN YOUR POTENTIAL

In which situation can you resolve an emotional dilemma by taking the time to understand the underlying cause of why you feel the way you do? Navigate this challenge by channelling your emotions rather than allowing yourself to be swept away by them.

Mountains and rivers in dreams represent challenges in your waking life that you can directly relate to. You may also dream that you have no obvious points of reference to guide you on your journey towards your deeper purpose.

Lost in a forest

UNLOCK THE MEANING

A forest symbolizes the unspoken and often unseen aspects of your purpose that are continually growing and maturing. Feeling lost indicates that you are becoming more aware of all the possibilities for your future healthy growth but are unsure how to make the most of your rich and varied inner resources.

AWAKEN YOUR POTENTIAL

Choose the way forward that feels instinctively right. As you do so, you will find new opportunities that will help keep you on the right path. Consider the occasions when you can be more open to exploring unfamiliar possibilities and where they might take you.

As you navigate different waking-life challenges, it can sometimes seem as if the purposeful path you are following is beginning to disappear with no obvious way forward.

Disappearing path

UNLOCK THE MEANING

Dreaming of a disappearing path reflects a situation in your waking life that you feel has served its purpose and can take you no further. Although you may feel that there is no way forward, this is your opportunity to break new ground and inspire others to follow in your footsteps.

AWAKEN YOUR POTENTIAL

Break away from the footsteps of others. Follow your own path in life by creating a clear vision of the direction you want to follow without losing sight of where you have come from. We can often feel that we have to follow the paths set out for us by others in order to be accepted, but following in the footsteps of others can leave us feeling that we are stuck in a rut. Although it may seem easier to follow an established route, such as a formalized career path, that can limit your choices and ability to develop your full potential. Creating your own trail in life requires more effort and will take you out of your comfort zone, but it is ultimately more rewarding.

Potential Dreams

As well as helping you to understand who you are and who you have been in your waking life, your dreams also help you to realize who you can become. Many of us feel that we have much greater potential than we are currently utilizing in our day-to-day lives but are unsure how to make the most of it. These feelings are reflected in dreams about our life potential. In these dreams, we often encounter situations in which opportunities should be opening up for us but, for some reason, nothing seems to be actually happening to help us reach our potential.

Broken-down car

UNLOCK THE MEANING

Dreaming of a broken-down car indicates a situation in your waking life in which you feel that you are finding it difficult to get fired up and motivated about a particular ambition. This can often be a result of realizing that reaching your full potential may require a long and arduous journey.

AWAKEN YOUR POTENTIAL

Ensure that you have all the resources you need to fuel your ambitions. This will help you maintain your momentum as you make steady progress towards fulfilling your potential. Like any driving force in your waking life, you have to nurture the things that motivate you in order to maintain forward motion. If you allow your energy to be dissipated by distractions, you will find it more difficult to focus your efforts on the specific outcome that you really want to achieve.

Feeling demotivated or realizing that it will take a long time to achieve your ambitions can make you concerned that you will miss an important opportunity to fulfil your potential. This can manifest in a dream where you are late for something.

Being late

UNLOCK THE MEANING

When you dream of being late, it reflects a situation in your waking life in which you feel that your time is not your own. This is often because you are spending much of your time helping other people to reach their potential and not devoting enough to fulfilling your own potential.

AWAKEN YOUR POTENTIAL

In which situations do you need to give yourself the time to do things that matter to you? Continue helping other people but make sure that you also take the time for yourself.

Reaching your potential requires you to maintain your momentum and make progress to a timetable of your own choosing. When you feel that you are learning how to reach your potential but have given yourself a deadline for doing so, you may find yourself dreaming about being back at school.

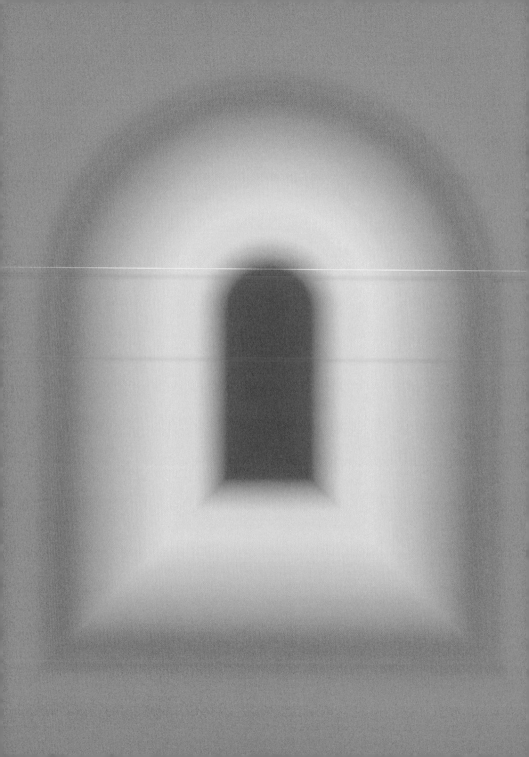

Back at school

UNLOCK THE MEANING

Dreaming of being back at school suggests that you have an opportunity in your waking life to learn more about yourself and how you can reach your full potential. Rather than learning about how other people have reached their goals, now is the time to gain a deeper understanding of how you can reach yours.

AWAKEN YOUR POTENTIAL

Instead of thinking that you are all you ever will be, make the commitment to being open to learning more about yourself. It can be tempting to ignore and skip important life lessons, but that can leave you with a very elementary understanding of who you are and how you relate to the world around you. Being receptive to gaining insights about yourself provides you with a higher degree of self-awareness and a healthy realization of what you can achieve in life.

When you dream of being unprepared for an exam, whether at school or at college, it suggests that you're attempting to judge yourself rather than trying to learn about your potential.

Unprepared for an exam

UNLOCK THE MEANING

Exams reflect how you assess your ability to achieve your potential in life. Dreaming of being unprepared for an exam indicates a situation in your waking life where you are critically examining your performance. In this case, you may think you should already have an answer for everything rather than being open to learning.

AWAKEN YOUR POTENTIAL

You may be familiar with being self-critical and never feeling good enough. Celebrate your achievements to date instead of subjecting yourself to endless self-examination about failing to fulfil your potential. Routinely judging yourself too harshly can leave you feeling that you will never achieve the goals you are pursuing in your life.

As well as pursuing an ambition, the word 'pursuit' can also be used in the context of being chased or chasing something, as in dreams where you are stalked by a monster.

Pursued by a monster

UNLOCK THE MEANING

When you dream of being chased by a monster, there is a situation in your waking life in which you have become aware of a monster opportunity to fulfil your potential. Your doubts about your ability to succeed with it, however, have grown out of all proportion and are in danger of becoming self-destructive.

AWAKEN YOUR POTENTIAL

In which cases might you be blowing your concerns out of proportion as you engage with a big opportunity? Have the confidence to turn the situation around so that you become the one who is pursuing the opportunity rather than feeling it is pursuing you.

It is only natural to try to hide from a scary pursuer, but hiding prevents any forward progress. This can result in a situation where you keep such a low profile that no one knows you are actually there.

Being invisible

UNLOCK THE MEANING

Dreaming of being invisible indicates a waking-life situation in which you feel that your potential is not being recognized by other people. Although you might blame others for not acknowledging your achievements, this often occurs because you feel that you may not live up to your own idealized self-image.

AWAKEN YOUR POTENTIAL

Confidently raise your profile and make your talent more visible to the people around you. Once aware of your achievements, they can appreciate your potential and help you develop it. When you feel invisible and keep a low profile, it can seem as if the image that you present to other people doesn't really matter. But this can also influence how you view yourself, so make sure you give yourself credit for your achievements.

As you take action to raise your profile, you will often find yourself in situations that may initially seem strange to you. Engaging with these unfamiliar situations will naturally surface your hidden potential and draw your attention to how you can use it effectively.

Stranger with a message

UNLOCK THE MEANING

When you dream of meeting a stranger who has a message for you, you are actually communicating the promise of your future development to yourself. That is because the stranger you meet in your dreams is actually that as-yet-unexplored part of yourself that holds all your future potential. Although you may think you know yourself very well, most of your self-awareness operates below the threshold of conscious thought in waking life. Your dreams actively process the rest of your self-awareness and express a wider and deeper awareness of who you have the potential to become.

AWAKEN YOUR POTENTIAL

Communicating with the person you have yet to become can be a strange experience, so be open to the messages you are sending yourself. These messages are often invitations to step into unknown and unfamiliar situations in your waking life that may seem quite strange to you at first. As you accept these invitations, you will often find yourself experiencing new and valuable aspects of who you are and what you can achieve.

FURTHER DREAM WORK

The images and emotions that you create in your dreams don't just disappear when you wake from your sleep. They continue to inhabit your unconscious awareness during the day and can be roused at any time you choose, so you can reconnect with their power. The easiest way to do this is through using dream work exercises, described in the following methods. These techniques naturally feed back into your night-time dreams in a very positive and healthy manner.

Love & Sex

It can be tempting to wish for a perfect lover who will see all the great qualities in you that you may not see yourself. Rather than waiting for that vision of perfection to arrive, you can make yourself more intimately aware of your admirable qualities and secret desires. Find a quiet and comfortable place where you will not be disturbed. Begin writing a love letter to yourself, as if you were your own secret admirer. This is not narcissism; it is simply giving yourself the opportunity to become more aware of the qualities you admire most in yourself. In your letter, share some examples of how you embody and express those qualities in your day-to-day life. Then write down a secret desire, such as an idea or a plan that you are very passionate about. Invite yourself to be your own companion and confidante in order to turn your secret desire into reality.

Relationships & Family

Although we may routinely describe ourselves as being of a specific age, we all embody a range of psychological ages, no matter how many years we have been alive. We all have a younger, more playful part of ourselves and an older, wiser part. Whatever age you currently are, take that number away from 100 and write down the result. If you are over 100 years old, then well done, and use 150 instead. If you are 50 or close to it, then imagine yourself as being significantly either younger or older. Otherwise, imagine yourself being the age of the number you have written down. Have an imaginary conversation with that person and ask them what advice they would give to you at your current age. Write down the piece of advice that resonates most strongly with you and reflect on how you might act on it.

Birth & Death

Find a gate or a doorway where you are free to step backwards and forwards through it. Make sure that you will not be disturbed and can spend the time you need. Designate one side of the opening as your future and the other side as your past. Begin on your past side and give yourself permission to step forward across the threshold into your future. As you do so, reflect on what you would like to welcome into your future and what you would like to let go of from your past. Step through your gate or doorway a few times to see what emerges and evolves for you. When you need to let go of the past to step into emerging opportunities, your biggest challenge can often be giving yourself permission to take the steps you need to move into the beckoning possibilities of your new future.

Work & Play

Two of the most highly prized professional skills are the ability to perform under pressure and the ability to create original solutions to complex problems. Being able to display your performance skills and showcase your talents will attract support for your abilities and ensure that you always succeed in any professional challenges. Imagine that your work environment is the venue for a unique form of sporting activity. That sport is the work that you routinely do on a day-to-day basis. Then imagine yourself as a television sports commentator describing your performance. Listen to yourself commentating on what you consider to be one of your unique talents in your working environment. Write down that unique talent and, as you do so, imagine a large crowd cheering you on. Then switch television channels and imagine yourself as the presenter of an arts programme, excitedly describing the originality and creativity that you bring to the work that you do.

Wealth & Health

In both wealth and health dreams, people are searching for what they value most. This exercise reflects that searching process in order to help bring a valuable realization to the surface. Get ready to go for a walk. Before you head outside for your walk, draw an outline of a treasure island on a sheet of paper. Close your eyes and mark an X on the paper inside the outline. Without looking at it, fold the paper up and put it in your pocket. Then go for a walk, and as you walk, imagine yourself strolling around the treasure island that you drew on the sheet of paper. Imagine yourself heading towards the X and, as you do so, ask yourself what you value most about yourself. When your answer emerges, unfold the paper and write it down beside the X.

Travel & Discovery

The route to achieving your aspirations and ambitions can often seem like uncharted territory and you may find yourself wishing that you had a native guide to steer you towards the outcome that you hope to arrive at. You can become your own guide by going for a walk for an hour or so in one of your favourite places, taking a notebook and pen with you. Imagine that you are the leader of an expedition to find a lost civilization. As you walk, let your mind wander and be open to observing details that you may have not noticed before or that perhaps seemed insignificant. Document these details by writing them down as you discover them. As you write each one down, write something special about yourself that you may not have noticed before or that perhaps seemed insignificant to you.

Purpose & Potential

Take yourself to a quiet place somewhere outside where you will not be disturbed. If you can, find a forest or wood to walk in. If not, go somewhere that is slightly unfamiliar but where you will feel comfortable and can safely return from. Stand in the centre of that place and start slowly turning around on the spot where you are standing. You will feel yourself wanting to stop at some point, so just let that happen. Then start walking forward and, as you do so, say to yourself 'My life purpose is...' and see what emerges for you. This exercise is about quietening the busy self-critical mind and allowing you to identify and focus on the direction you want to take in life by intuitively seeing what emerges from your unconscious.

MAKE YOUR DREAMS COME TRUE

Working with your night-time dreams is one of the most natural and healthy ways to develop your self-awareness and situational awareness. As you develop these, you often become more aware of opportunities to use your power and achieve your ambitions in your waking life. Making your dreams come true isn't simply a matter of wishing them into existence. Instead, it's a process of asking yourself the questions and taking the actions that emerge from your dreams. Let's look at some practical ways of how to do that in this chapter.

Remembering Your Dreams

A basic requirement for decoding dreams is actually being able to remember the imagery that you created as you were dreaming. Quite often, people will firmly declare that they never dream. In reality, though, all human beings dream for around two hours a night. People who say that they never dream just don't remember the dreams that they create. There are a range of reasons why you might not remember your dreams and these include the brain's memory consolidation process, the threshold effect and physically moving your body as soon as you wake up.

One of the functions of dreaming is to consolidate your meaningful memories by processing them from your short-term memory into long-term memory. This memory consolidation process means that it can be challenging to recall what is actually happening in your dream. It's like trying to record some music or video but also trying to play it back at the same time. The threshold effect describes the way your attention shifts when you move across the threshold between one attention space and another. It's as if you are in one room in waking life and decide that you need to get something from another room. When you walk across the threshold into the other room, the change in attention space can make you forget what it is that you needed in that room.

'Will, Still, Fill' Method

As soon as you start moving your body when you wake, your dream imagery starts to fade away. The easiest way to recall your dreams is to remember three words, which are **WILL**, **STILL** and **FILL**:

As you settle down to sleep at night, say to yourself 'Tonight I **WILL** remember my dreams.'

When you wake up, just lie completely **STILL** for a minute. Don't move your body, don't even wiggle your toes.

As you lie still, images and emotions from your dreams will emerge for you. Then **FILL** in the gaps between the dream images and you will naturally begin to remember your dream.

Recording Your Dreams

One of the best ways to remember your dreams consistently is to write them down in a dream diary. Although dreams can seem to be one-off events, keeping a dream diary often reveals deeper patterns in your dream themes and shows you how they are developing over time. The documented evidence of your dreams in a dream diary is a great self-development resource because it enables you to pose yourself questions and coach yourself through them. Writing down your dreams in your dream diary is also a very useful way of engaging with what you are trying to communicate to yourself in recurring dreams.

There are a wide range of methods for keeping a dream diary and there is no one best method for everyone. The best method for you is the one that suits you and your circumstances. My favourite method is to use a dedicated notebook that I keep beside my bed. Another option is having a voice-activated recorder beside your bed, although this makes it difficult to search through your narrations of what you experienced in your dreams. An increasingly popular method is using your phone to record a selfie video describing your dream and then transcribing that into a notebook later.

For the notebook method, I quickly write down imagery and emotions from the dream on the left-hand page of two facing pages. I don't try to analyze the dream at this point but just jot down everything I can remember about the dream. Some details may seem insignificant at the time, but they can often reveal a deeper meaning on further reflection. I describe the dream in the present tense to retain its immediacy as that makes it easier to re-engage with later. As my dream notebook is a diary, I write the date for each entry so I can chart the progression of the dream imagery that I am creating.

Then later on, I come back to what I wrote and use the right-hand page to decode the dream and understand it in more depth. I work through the left-hand page and identify characters, places, events and objects that seemed to have significance. I usually sketch these out on the right-hand page and explore anything that might connect them. Memory works by association, so making these connections often triggers new insights. As I work through the dream imagery and potential connections, I am usually beginning to form a hypothesis, as described in 'Decoding Your Dreams' (see pages 25–27), so I write my hypothesis at the top of the right-hand page.

After writing down my hypothesis, I look through my notes, sketches and reflections so far to see if they still support that hypothesis. If they do, I write down a meaning for the dream, then note down the action that has emerged from decoding the dream. After noting down the action, I write down the question that will help me take the action from the dream into my waking life. Recording your dreams using a dream diary in this way doesn't need to be a lengthy or overinvolved process. Simply take as long as you need to play around with the imagery that you created.

Influencing Your Dreams

Although you actively create your dreams, it may sometimes seem like you are a passive observer and you might wish that you could somehow influence your dreams and the content that you create in them. There are three main approaches that you can use to influence your dream content. The first of these is making the choice to create an appropriate sleeping environment, the second is choosing what you eat and drink before you go to bed and the third is the phenomenon of lucid dreaming. Working with these three approaches will help you to influence your dream content and quality.

The better your sleep quality, the better the quality of your dreams, so make your bedroom a cool, dark haven where you can sleep undisturbed for as long as you need. Remove all nonessential electronic equipment, such as televisions, computers and phones. This might stop you from overstimulating your brain before you go to sleep. There is a popular misconception that cheese causes nightmares. The reality is that eating any hard-to-digest food before you go to bed, such as cheese or a spicy curry, will result in your digestive system being highly active when you're trying to relax and go to sleep. As this will disturb your sleep patterns, you are more likely to wake up and your dream content may be more disturbing.

Alcohol is sometimes used as a way of relaxing before you go to sleep, and although it has some sedative properties to begin with, it becomes a stimulant as your body processes it and that may cause you to become wide awake after only a few hours of sleep. So cutting back on alcohol can also be a helpful idea.

The most powerful way to influence your dreams is to develop your capacity for lucid dreaming. This is the ability to become aware that you are dreaming while you're still asleep, and then using that awareness to consciously influence your dream content without waking yourself up.

Choosing Your Dreams

It used to be thought that dreams happened to us, but as we now know, we create our dreams. One of the reasons for thinking that dreams happened to us is that we seem to have very little control over the dream images and themes that we experience when we sleep. It also was once thought that waking and dreaming were two mutually exclusive states of awareness, but we now know that it is possible to realize that you are dreaming without immediately waking from the dream. This unique state of awareness, of being conscious that you are dreaming, is known as lucid dreaming.

Lucid dreaming is sometimes considered to be quite challenging to attain. Conventional methods of learning to lucid dream often seem to involve having to follow particular spiritual beliefs or using various types of electronic gadgets. The reality, however, is that all human beings have a natural talent for lucid dreaming and actually do it very briefly at least twice a night. The first time is as you are falling asleep. You may be thinking about the day's experiences and tomorrow's expectations, when an unconscious image will suddenly emerge into your consciousness. This is known as the hypnagogic phase.

The other time usually occurs less suddenly and that is when you are waking up. Our sleep cycles progress in such a way that we usually wake from a dream and there will be a point, just as you are waking up, where you are conscious that you are dreaming. This phase is known as the hypnopompic. Both the hypnagogic and hypnopompic phases provide you with the opportunity to play around with the unconscious dream imagery that you are creating. The ability to manipulate your dream imagery is known as ludic dreaming and is a natural companion to lucid dreaming.

The first step in learning to lucid dream consistently is simply observing that you are creating unconscious imagery. To begin with, that observation might last for a fleeting moment before you fall asleep or wake up. You will find that the more often you actively observe your unconscious imagery, the longer you can make the experience last. The next step is to start changing the imagery that you are creating. For example, if the image of a tree emerges from your unconscious, try making it taller or smaller. Then try making it brighter green or darker green. Try making it closer to you or further away from you.

By giving yourself the skill to play around with your unconscious imagery, you naturally start to develop the ability to make choices in your dreams. At first, this will mainly be in the hypnagogic and hypnopompic phases. The more that you do it, the more other opportunities to do it will emerge in your deeper dreams. One of the best times to practise lucid dreaming is quite counter-intuitive and that's because it is when you are creating the experience of a nightmare. Dreams and nightmares are often considered to be separate phenomena, but a nightmare is just a dream that is more emotionally powerful and intense.

Apart from their emotional potency, a key feature of many nightmares is that you become aware that you are creating a nightmare and so you try to wake yourself up from it. At that point, you have a choice. You can wake yourself up or you can engage with your dream imagery and work with it. For example, if you are being chased by a monster, make it smaller, make it friendlier or make it help you in the dream. You might also ask it who it is and what it needs. As you do so, you will begin a powerful conversation with your inner self.

When you actively engage with some aspect of a dream, you are actually engaging with a deeper, wiser part of yourself. Although it might seem scary and unsettling, you are acknowledging that you sometimes need to step outside your comfort zone to make the most of your potential. The more that you engage with the unspoken parts of your potential, the more likely you are to succeed in whatever waking-life challenges you encounter. Using lucid dreaming to make powerful and healthy choices in your dreams also makes you far more aware that you have the capacity to make powerful and healthy choices in your waking life.

Quick Dream Decoding Guide

Give yourself the opportunity to create high-quality dreams by creating high-quality sleep. Ensure that it is dark and cool in your bedroom, with minimal distractions, particularly from electronic media.

————————○————————

Remember your dreams by using the 'will, still, and fill' technique (see page 177). Keep a record of your dreams by creating a dream diary. Look for overall patterns emerging from a series of dreams as well as in individual dreams.

————————○————————

As you reflect on the imagery that you created in your dream, form a hypothesis of what it might mean. Explore how your dream imagery supports your hypothesis and identify the meaning that feels right for you.

————————○————————

A dream is just a dream until you put it into action, so choose the action that you are communicating to yourself in the dream. Ask yourself the question that will help you put your dream into action.

FURTHER READING

Blechner, Mark J., *The Dream Frontier*, Routledge, 2014

Damasio, Antonio, *The Feeling Of What Happens: Body, Emotion and the Making of Consciousness*, Vintage, 2000

Geary, James, *I Is an Other: The Secret Life of Metaphor and How it Shapes the Way We See the World*, Harper Collins, 2011

Lakoff, George and Mark Johnson, *Metaphors We Live By*, University of Chicago Press, 2003

Lakoff, George, '**Metaphor: The Language of the Unconscious – The Theory of Conceptual Metaphor Applied to Dream Analysis**', *IASD*, 1992

Laureys, Steven and Giulio Tononi, *The Neurology of Consciousness: Cognitive Neuroscience and Neuropathology*, Academic Press, 2011

Nir, Yuval and Giulio Tononi, '**Dreaming and the Brain: from Phenomenology to Neurophysiology**', *Trends in Cognitive Sciences* 14 (2):88-100, 2010

Piaget, Jean, *Play, Dreams and Imitation in Childhood*, Routledge, 2013

Solms, Mark, *The Neuropsychology of Dreams: A Clinico-Anatomical Study*, Routledge, 2015

Wallace, Ian, *The Complete A to Z Dictionary of Dreams: Be Your Own Dream Expert*, Vermillion, 2014

Wallace, Ian, *The Top 100 Dreams: The Dreams That We All Have and What They Really Mean*, Hay House, 2011

Winget, Carolyn and Milton Kramer, *Dimensions of Dreams*, University Press of Florida, 1979

Index

About the Author

I am endlessly curious about human nature and why people do the things that they do. That's why I became a psychologist: to understand human behaviour, particularly in complex high-consequence situations.

I have worked professionally on a North Sea oil rig, as a mountain guide, session musician, fashion photographer, commercial pilot, military psychologist, relationship counsellor, child psychologist, celebrity psychologist and technology entrepreneur. Although these may appear to be quite diverse, they are united by my fundamental fascination with human nature and my continuing research into how people find meaning, purpose and potential in the work that they do.

The work I do with dreams forms a fundamental part of my psychology practice. It has proven to be one of the healthiest and most natural ways of developing those human superpowers of self-awareness and situational awareness. It is focused on the practical application of our night-time dreams as a positive and healthy method to help us achieve our waking-life dreams and ambitions.

This practical approach has led to regular appearances on television and radio around world, and becoming the best-selling author of *The Top 100 Dreams: The Dreams That We All Have and What They Really Mean* and *The Complete A to Z Dictionary of Dreams: Be Your Own Dream Expert.*

ianwallacedreams.com

Acknowledgements

A massive thank you to the fantastic editorial and design team of Zara Anvari, Laura Bulbeck, Jessica Axe, Isabel Eeles, and Michelle Kliem at White Lion Publishing.

A huge appreciation to all my fabulous TV and radio Dream Apprentices, Greg James, Gemma Collins, Scarlett Moffatt, Ryan Seacrest, Jim Jefferies, Forrest Shaw, Kelly Blackheart, Jack Hackett, Eleri Sion, Jeremy Vine, Phillip Schofield, Holly Willoughby, Mollie King, Matt Edmondson, Eamonn Holmes, Ruth Langsford, Joey Page, Russell Brand, Rylan Clark-Neal, Ben Shephard, Kelsey Patel, Ryan Patrick Hooper, Amanda LeClaire, Sarah Jeynes, Tim Smith and Steve Wright, for the opportunity to explore the awesome dreams of our viewers and listeners.

First published in 2021 by White Lion Publishing,
an imprint of The Quarto Group.
The Old Brewery, 6 Blundell Street
London, N7 9BH,
United Kingdom
T (0)20 7700 6700
www.QuartoKnows.com

A catalogue record for this book is available from the British Library.

ISBN 978 0 7112 5705 4
Ebook ISBN 978 0 7112 5706 1

10 9 8 7 6 5 4 3 2 1

Publisher   Jessica Axe
Commissioning Editor   Zara Anvari
Senior Editor   Laura Bulbeck
Art Direction   Isabel Eeles
Design   Michelle Kliem

Printed in China

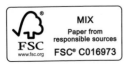